It Smells Just Like Popcorn

The Modern Woman's A to V Guide to Her Vagina and Beyond

The New Edition

Dr. Wendy Goodall McDonald

Dr. Every Woman

Edited by Rae Lynne Johnson

Cover Art by Rahsaan Taylor

Cover Photo by Anthony Rose Photography

Dr. Every Woman Publishing

200 S. Michigan Ave, Suite 1550

Chicago, IL, 60604

www.dreverywoman.com

ISBN: 978-0-9993341-2-6

DEDICATION

I dedicate this book to my family, both blood and otherwise, and to my mentor, Dr. Lewanzer Lassiter, the woman who showed me who I could be.

CONTENTS

DISCLAIMER

The content in this book is for informational purposes only. This book should not be used as a substitute for medical advice from your own physician. You should never delay seeking medical care and advice, disregard medical care and advice, or commence or discontinue any medical care or treatment because of information in this book. If you have questions on the topics discussed in this book, you should consult your physician.

Every effort has been made to make this book as complete and accurate as possible. However, there may be mistakes both typographical and in content. Therefore, this text should be used only as a general guide and not as an ultimate source of medical information. Furthermore, this book contains information current only up to the printing date.

The purpose of this book is to inform and to help. The author and publisher shall have neither liability nor responsibility to any person or entity with respect to any loss or damage caused, or alleged to be caused, directly or indirectly by the information contained in this book.

FOREWORD
BY DR. SHELLY AGARWAL FROM THE GYNECO-(B)LOGIC

What a daunting task it can be to learn about the human body. We all have one, and yet the intricacies often evade most of us. One of my most vivid memories is when I went to a friend's place for a book club. The company was made up of fairly educated and professional women – lawyers, teachers, doctors. When they found out that I was an OB/GYN, the onslaught of questions started.

"My Pap was abnormal. Does that mean I may have uterine cancer?" ("No, it doesn't.")
"Wait, so what's bacterium vaginitisosis?" ("Not a real diagnosis.")
"Wait. Wait. Wait. What's a cervix?"

I couldn't believe it. I knew that women's health and anatomy were taboo topics for many women, but I never realized just how little we know about our lady bits, and what the implications are when something goes wrong. Often the majority of my office visits are filled with not only educating women about their body parts, but also dispelling myths and falsehoods they have picked up during their lives, not only from Dr. Google but also from their aunt's hairdresser's best friend's cousin's mother who read an article in Reader's Digest once in the '80s. It can be dangerous, because not only does miseducation lead to improper self-treatment of common ailments, but also because it can cause women to ignore serious health concerns or symptoms that should be addressed.

Dr. Wendy Goodall McDonald and I have known each other for close to a decade. In that time we have weathered residency, boards, private practice and writing a blog together. I not only consider her a colleague, but also a close friend, who shares the same passion for empowerment through education for women of all ages. When she told me that she was writing a book on common gynecologic facts and diagnoses, a road map through the uterus, ovaries, cervix, vagina and vulva, I was ecstatic.

Finally, a resource from a trusted source that women can turn to as a precursor and addition to their Gyne visits! She's so darn funny while she teaches, too! I have thoroughly I enjoyed reading this book, and I am not too proud to say that I learned a thing or two.

May your vagina stay happy, healthy and pH balanced.

—Dr. Shelly Agarwal

INTRODUCTION: POPCORN, THE NEW EDITION

What does your vagina smell like?

Oh, sorry. I meant to ease you into this book. That was too much too soon. Let's try this, does your vagina smell like popcorn? Whether your answer is yes, or no, you've come to the right place because it smells like something.

This book is for every woman who has ever wondered about her body. Is my discharge normal? What should my vagina look like? Should I leak urine when I laugh? How do I stop that? Oh, you're too young for that last one? You just wait. I am going to help you understand your body, as well as help you solve many common gynecologic problems and prevent many others. You need to know these pearls, and so does your friend, sister, partner, cousin, play cousin and everyone else with or without a vagina. (I'm an equal opportunity health educator.)

In my Gyne practice (pronounced Guy-Knee. Please don't call me a Gyno. It's not derogatory, I just don't like the way that it sounds. It's like when someone calls you the wrong nickname) women come to see me for routine health maintenance and to solve health-related problems. The majority of my visits are with women who seek understanding about what is happening in their bodies. Well, ladies, this one is for you. I put together a list of every women's health topic that I could think of and answers to every question I am regularly asked. My patients often tell me that I break down topics in a way that helps them understand better than ever before. In this book I expand that breakdown beyond my office.

Would you buy a nice new techy device and not educate yourself about how to care for it? No. You would want to protect your investment by being informed. It is for this reason that I became a gynecologist. Even as a young girl, I sought to understand why every time I took a bubble bath, my girly parts were irritated and uncomfortable. It took my best friend's mother, who was an OB/GYN, to bring light to the fact that not all women can expose every product to their girlies. The delicate part of me was not interested in the fact that this body wash made pink bubbles and let me draw pictures with it on my washcloth. She was irritated by that cute wash, literally.

I actually knew that I wanted to be a gynecologist at an early age. Weird concept? Sure. Many children will say in the cutest of kid voices that they want to be a doctor, or a nurse, or a lawyer, or an astronaut. How many 5-year-olds can pronounce, let alone aspire to be, gynecologists? If you ask my dad, that was little Wendy Goodall (or "Sweets", as he still calls me because of my love for all things sugary). The desire was partially selfish in that I felt that if I knew about this bubble bath madness now, how much more womanly information could I learn to keep myself healthy and comfortable?

Sorry, men. Apart from being a circumcision expert (yes, that is a thing), I can't help you guys with your parts. The exception to that statement is that if I can help the women in your life be healthier, maybe they will also be happier, and you will be the beneficiaries of that happiness. By beneficiary, I mean that she could do something nice for you or smile a little more, or not be as mean or grumpy. If your mind automatically went between the "sheets", get that mind out of the gutter.

This book will not teach you how to do what I do, but it will give you a window into my world. Some basic truths about health can save you from unfortunate outcomes or at the very least, lend understanding where it is lacking. Not every OB/GYN can sit and talk to you for 20 minutes about your abnormal Pap test or why you may have discharge. That's what THIS BOOK is for!

To the mothers or mature women thinking about giving a copy of this book to your daughter or a young woman in your life, DO IT! Misinformation is so prevalent. I can't tell you how many people don't know how STI/STDs are transmitted, which ones are dangerous, that pull-out is an unreliable form of birth control, that the clap is not chlamydia (it is actually gonorrhea), and that a person doesn't need to have a lot of sex to get pregnant. It just takes once.

If you give your kid a car and some car keys but don't give him or her driving lessons or education on the rules of the road, eventually they may learn how to start the car on their own, or their friends will teach them. Pause and imagine that your kid's body is the car and puberty is the key. At some point, they will likely put that car into gear and try to drive. They will probably run into some things, blow through some traffic signals and get some tickets. Let's pray they don't hurt themselves or anyone else. Instead, if you teach them about the car and give them reasons why they might not want to drive yet, they might make wiser decisions.

I posed the following question to a teen in my practice who was sexually active but was reluctant to have STD testing or to start using reliable birth control because she didn't want her mother to know what she was doing. I asked her, "Which do you think your mother would dislike more: Finding out that you are having sex, but knowing that you are trying to be as safe as possible, or not knowing that you are having sex and as a result, you contract an undiagnosed STD or unplanned pregnancy?" I have a daughter. I would prefer for her to not have sex until she is either married or at least mentally prepared for the emotional weight that it carries. Damn a hookup! Trust and believe, though, that she will be well informed AND know that she can always talk to me or ask me questions, regardless of whether I agree with her decision.

Enjoy my A to Z indexed guide to all things female. I realize that my title says A-V, and no, that is not a typo. It was just catchier than A-Z. Far be it from me to leave out W, X, Y and Z in this book.

Here's an important notice: Now that we've discussed what this book is, let's briefly discuss what this book isn't. This book does not create a doctor-patient relationship between me (the author) and you (the reader). While I am a doctor, I'm not your doctor. That means you should not wait to seek treatment from your doctor, start or stop any prescribed medical treatment, or disregard your doctor's advice based on what you read here. I'm here to educate you, not to treat you. That's an important distinction. Also, to the extent that I include links or references or other sources, they are for your information only, not an endorsement on my part of any product or content. #legalese #CYA

Throughout the book, there will be many more disclaimers, along with hashtags, and parenthetical remarks. It is the state of my brain. Just bear with me. #iknowhashtagsdontworkinbooks
In the words of the hilarious comedian, Tiffany Haddish, "She READY!"

Also, for the non-binary, please excuse the extensive use of pronouns in this book. Feel free to insert your pronoun of choice where you deem appropriate. My pronouns are She, Her, and Hers. Thank you.

1
POPCORN

"So, what brings you in today?"

"Well, Doc, I have been noticing a new smell from (gesturing) down there, and I don't know what it is or why it is there."

"How long have you noticed it?"

"I don't know, maybe a week or two."

"Okay, well, does it itch or burn or anything?"

"No."

"Any new sexual partners or unprotected sex?"

"No."

"Hmm. What does it smell like?"

"It...it kind of smells like popcorn."

"Like popcorn?" Throat clears to hide the involuntary chuckle. "What kind of popcorn? I mean, this is a first. I've never heard this before. I'm not sure what to ask."

"Well, I Googled it (fingernails on a chalkboard) and it seems kind of common."

"Really? Popcorn?"

"Yes. Buttered, non-buttered, people who eat popcorn, people who don't..."

"Do you eat popcorn?"

"Sometimes."

"What did the Google ladies say was the cause?"

"They didn't know, but they knew it smelled like popcorn."

Popcorn. By far the most profoundly entertaining noun I have ever heard to describe the smell exuding from a person's vagina. I literally could not hold back my chuckle-smile combination. Imagine this moment. "Doc, my vagina has a smell." Me: "What does it smell like? Fishy? Pungent?" My differential diagnosis (a hypothetical list of possible things that could be causing the problem) is possibly bacterial vaginosis, or the dreaded retained tampon that has been out of my patient's reach for days to weeks. It could also be yeast, which infrequently causes odor, but can. "Popcorn." (snort, snicker, sniff) "Popcorn?"

"Yes, like popcorn. I don't even eat popcorn but that is literally what it smells like."

I send a panel of tests for various vaginal infections. Then I pay Google a visit, just because. I find pages and pages of women describing their vaginas as buttered, and unbuttered, sweet, yellow, cheesy, "I eat popcorn," "I don't even eat popcorn," and so on and so forth. I literally cannot believe how many women are writing about this subject and I am entertained as hell. Let's tackle this and many other medical aspects head on. Then we can read posts and articles about popcorn for their entertainment value, without having to really believe that Orville Redenbacher paid our "business" a visit. I'm going to start calling mine Chicago Mix. (Get at me Garrett's. This is an ad campaign you can't pass up.)

A.

Abstinence
Find this topic under contraceptives.

"I can't overwhelm you with all of my game. I have to conserve my game. "

- Mos Def, Brown Sugar

Ablation
See Hysteroscopy. Don't worry. I won't be doing this for the whole book.

Acne/Androgens

Acne can be caused by many things, including excess testosterone or testosterone-like hormones known as androgens. Adolescence leads to a whole host of hormone surges that can make a face look like pepperoni pizza. Acne can be normal, but sometimes it is a sign of an underlying problem.

Acne caused by hormonal imbalance can occur when a person has a thyroid issue or ovulation dysfunction, to give a couple of examples. If a woman's periods are inconsistent, too frequent or too infrequent, and this is coupled with acne problems, hormonal abnormalities could be to blame. Menstrual cycles that are more than 35 days apart (without a pregnancy) or less than 21 days apart (again without a pregnancy) are classified as abnormal. We count from day 1 of the menstrual cycle to the next day 1 to determine the duration. Also, if one's period is 25 days apart, the next period is 35 days apart, the next is 21 days and so on, that isn't normal. Polycystic ovarian syndrome (PCOS) is a syndrome where ovarian dysfunction can lead to period irregularity, weight gain, acne and even fertility issues. More on this topic in the PCOS section. There I will discuss ways to diagnose and tackle androgen dysfunction.

Birth control pills are commonly used to improve acne. This is because they balance the hormonal fluctuations that can lead to acne. Yes, this is a temporary fix, but in medicine you learn that everything in our bodies doesn't always work perfectly so sometimes you need to manage symptoms. If you don't want to put a proverbial Band-Aid on this problem, just rock your acne with pride.

The acne take-home message is this: if over the counter facial cleansers aren't doing the trick, it may be time for a visit to the dermatologist or gynecologist or both, especially if menstrual cycle irregularities are present.

Alzheimer's

See Dementia.

Anatomy

Ahhh, here we go. The meat and potatoes! This is where the money is. Okay, sorry, here we go. I'm just so excited.

It's about time that we talk about anatomy. A good friend told me that her daughter was reprimanded in kindergarten because she said that she knew her mom was pregnant with a girl because the ultrasound showed a vagina instead of a penis. She was reprimanded for saying the words "vagina" and "penis" in kindergarten. I LOVE that a 6-year-old knew the proper terminology and could say it without giggling. Now you say it with me, VA-GI-NA.

A study of British and US women showed that 44-80% of women were unable to locate parts of their anatomy in a drawing. The vagina, uterus, fallopian tubes, ovaries and vulva all stumped a large proportion of women. I can only hope that those same women could at least locate their vaginas on themselves. It would be crazy to think otherwise, except that I knew of a married couple who were unable to get pregnant. After very detailed and explicit questioning, it was discovered that anal sex had been their customary practice rather than just an adventurous one. Neither of them realized where her actual vagina was, or how to use it. No judgment against couples who are into that, but you can't get pregnant that way. There is no uterus in the anus/rectum. For some, that is part of their motivation.

My absolute favorite anatomy story of all time, at least so far, occurred on a quiet winter/spring day in Chicago. For those unfamiliar with Chicago climate, winter/spring represents the time of the year when it is spring by seasonal definition and chronology, but it is still very cold outside. Fall/winter and winter/spring are seasons that I have decided exist in the Chi. Anyway, a patient in her mid-forties was in my office to see me for her annual exam. As with all of my new and established patients, I asked her if she had any concerns that day.

"Well doc, I found a new bump down there. I am actually not sure how new it is. I never noticed it before and I was hoping you could check it out."

"Does it hurt? Does it come and go?"

"No, it doesn't hurt. I haven't noticed it changing. I just don't know what it is."

Running through my mind are things like an ingrown hair, a Bartholin gland cyst, an atypical herpes outbreak, a sebaceous cyst... the list goes on and on. The section in this book on "Things" goes into the many things a thing down there could be.

We proceed to chat through her annual exam as I check her out from head to toe, or more like neck to buttocks in my realm. We finish the exam and she sits back up. It dawns on me, what about that bump?

"I didn't see anything out of the ordinary down there."

"Well it is pretty big, can I point it out for you?"

"Sure."

Any guesses on where her finger pointed next? It was none other than her clitoris. Her CLIT-oris or her clit-TORIS. Either pronunciation will do the trick. Enlightening her to this magical anatomic discovery truly made my day. She was so embarrassed, but I assured her that I have seen worse on the lack of anatomy knowledge side of life. She was very grateful to have now discovered such a special part of her body. I don't want to know exactly how grateful she was. I can only hope for her sake that this was only the beginning of her discovery of the magical abilities of this little organ.

The clitoris is the epicenter of nerve endings for the female sex organs. It actually looks a lot like a small penis when visualized in its entirety. This is not surprising since men and women are formed of the same basic building blocks. The part of the clitoris that can be seen externally is only a small part – a true tip of the iceberg. The stimulation of the glans clitoris can lead to an orgasm. Some women are able to achieve an orgasm with direct stimulation. Some women are able to have an orgasm during penetrative intercourse and via indirect stimulation (motion in the ocean). Regardless of how an individual gets their jollies, this is an important place for most women in the arena of orgasms.

Outside of the sex discussion, the clitoris can also be a place of interest in countries where genital mutilation is still practiced. This practice can involve removal of all or part of the clitoral hood, the glans itself, the inner or outer labia, etc. The idea is to control female sexuality by altering a woman's anatomy. There are organizations where you can donate to increase education and hopefully stop these practices that can lead to dangerous bleeding, chronic pain, infections and difficulty with childbearing.

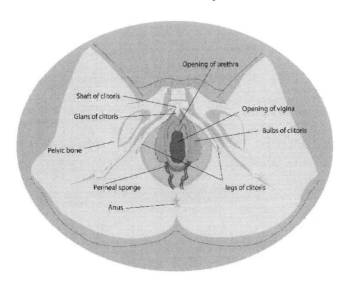

Female reproductive system

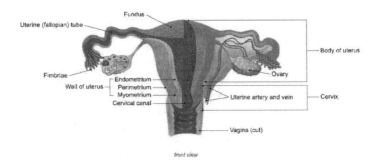

There are three holes.

The vagina is the opening that is located between where you urinate and where you have a bowel movement. This is where blood comes from during a period. The deepest part of the vagina also houses the cervix, which is the opening of the uterus. This is important because vagina intercourse with a penis can lead to pregnancy if the uterus and ovaries and fallopian tubes are present. It only takes one little lonely sperm, even if without ejaculation (or cum, to be crass) to sneak through that cervix, and unite with an egg. When the one egg and one sperm unite, a little life can be formed. If there are two eggs present, twins begin. If one egg and one sperm unite and split into two separate embryos, twins form as well. The point is that only a dab of sperm will do ya.

Because of this math (egg plus sperm equals baby), some believe that anal intercourse is valid contraception. Well, it is true that pregnancy will not occur with anal intercourse. Sexually transmitted diseases (STD), however, are still very easily transmitted. STD transmission is more likely with anal intercourse because the glands for lubrication are not present in the anus. Less lubrication can lead to small tears in the tissue can allow infections to creep in. Anal intercourse may be a back door to avoid pregnancy, but it isn't an easy way out (snicker snicker #punlife).

The vulva is defined as the female external genitalia. This includes the labia majora and the labia minora (the outer and inner lips), the opening of the vagina, the urethra and the perineum (the tissue between the vagina and the anus). What is important to realize about the vulva, and especially the labia, is that every woman's vulva is different. One of my favorite pieces of art was featured in the Huffington Post a few years back. It was called The Great Wall of Vagina. This artist cast in plaster the external genitalia of four hundred women. It is like looking at 400 fingerprints of not-the-finger. More on that in the Labia section.

The urethra is where the urine comes out. By urine, I mean pee. Hey, don't judge. We're breaking stuff down over here. You might catch me saying "poop" later on. I will NOT say "boo-boo" though. #Ijustsaidit. Your kidneys filter blood to remove excess water, imbalanced electrolytes, and other toxins or waste. That filtration produces urine. It passes out of the kidneys into tubes called ureters which empty into the bladder. When the bladder gets full enough, it signals to your brain that you have to "go." When you give the green light (or maybe the yellow light), you urinate out of the urethra. The urinary tract should be sterile, meaning bacteria-free. This is why wiping from front to back is so important. If you wipe from back to front, you are dragging vaginal and anal bacteria to the urethra, which can increase your chances for developing an infection.

The uterus is where babies can form, where blood sheds out, where an IUD can live, and where fibroids and polyps can grow.

11

The uterus has so much potential, both good and bad. When the uterus misbehaves, atypical tissue can form. This tissue can become cancerous if unchecked. For this reason, cycle irregularities should be evaluated by a doctor.

The cervix is like the main entrance to the uterus. It is where a Pap test and some STD tests are performed. It is supposed to stay closed until a pregnancy leads to labor and it opens. If it opens too soon during pregnancy, sometimes medication is required. Sometimes stitching it closed is necessary. It is a complex structure.

Touching the cervix isn't like touching your skin. Taking a cervical biopsy may feel like cramping rather than sharp pain. I make this point for the women who think they don't need a Pap or to see their Gyne because they would "know" if they had any cervical abnormalities. Cervical abnormalities are often silent. You usually don't feel them or have any symptoms, with the exception of abnormal bleeding, sometimes.

If the cervix is the front door of the uterus, the fallopian tubes are the back doors. They are the conduits for sperm and fertilized egg transfer. They can house infections like chlamydia and can lead to pelvic inflammatory disease. They can be full of fluid, which is called hydrosalpinx. They can be disconnected and tied for birth control — a permanent procedure called a tubal ligation. They cannot be reliably "untied." The risk of ectopic pregnancy is high. This is why I am anti-tubal ligation unless you are 110% SURE that you don't want any more kids. After a tubal ligation, in vitro fertilization (IVF) is your best bet to try to conceive.

The fallopian tubes are used as a conduit or track for transport of the ovulated or released egg to the inside of the uterus. The ovary releases the egg. The fallopian tube then vacuums it up and sends the egg toward the uterus.

Little known fallopian tube facts:
1.   Conception (fertilization of an egg by sperm) occurs in the tube, not in the uterus. Then, the embryo (the early cell-stage baby) continues its transport through this fleshy tube to later implant in the uterus.
2.   An embryo that gets stuck in the fallopian tube, or anywhere outside of the uterus, is called an ectopic pregnancy. In the event that this happens, treatment can include medication or surgery. Read all about ectopic pregnancies in the Ectopic Section.

3. Ovarian cancer arises mostly from ovarian cells, but science suggests that the fallopian tube can house cells that can become ovarian cancer as well. Because of this, the traditional tubal ligation for permanent contraception/sterilization is slowly being replaced with a salpingectomy or fallopian tube-ectomy, complete removal of the fallopian tube. The theory is that if you aren't going to use them anyway, why leave them there just to potentially cause trouble. That would be like finishing your summer barbeque, but instead of throwing your leftovers away, you just leave them to roast in the sun and attract flies. Okay, so these two scenarios are very dissimilar, but roll with it to get the point.

The anus is where you have bowel movements, or poop. One of my favorite comedians, Tiffany Haddish, referred to this location in the comedic blockbuster movie, Girls Trip, as "the booty hole." I think that the exact line was, "You can't get an infection in your booty hole. It's your booty hole!" How, you may ask, do I plan to turn this sidebar into an educational moment? Well, my only point, other than shouting out Tiffany Haddish (#iloveyou #getatme) is that you CAN get an infection in your anus. A rectal abscess is a "thing." Don't put objects in your "booty hole." It is not a pocket, a secret compartment, or a travel belt. There is ALWAYS a better place to put something.

The hymen is the tissue that is present at the opening of the vagina that serves as nature's chastity belt. That actually isn't true at all, the chastity belt part, that is. For some women, it makes the opening of the vagina small in caliber. It may even tear/break during initial penetrative intercourse. Once it is torn, it won't obstruct the vagina anymore, but the initial tear can be somewhat painful. I have had to open a woman's hymen surgically a few times because it either had no opening, or the opening was so small, that penetration or even tampon use was nearly impossible. A woman who cannot have intercourse, cannot use tampons, and cannot even get her own finger into her vagina raises suspicion for having an imperforate, or completely closed hymen. That is not the only possibility, but it is a likely one. Ultrasound or MRI is sometimes necessary to determine why the vagina isn't opened. A woman's medical history and physical exam will guide me to try to remove the "closed for renovations" sign on her vagina.

Within our ovaries, from the time of birth, live all of the

eggs we will ever have. Actually, millions of eggs are lost before we are even born. The number of eggs lost total almost as many revisions this book went through before going to print. Men have the luxury of making new sperm every day. We women have aging eggs that can start to malfunction over time like my 1990 Honda Accord right before I got a "new" used car in 2009. There is no mechanic for the ovaries. The closest things that we have are Reproductive Endocrinology and Infertility specialists, also known as REI doctors. They can sometimes help.

The ever-elusive G-spot. Get your tear-ready facial tissues out for this one. There is no proven anatomic location that is definite for the existence of the G-spot. I'm imagining a bunch of sex therapists and Karma Sutra experts chasing me with S&M whips and chains (not that I think that is something those groups would have, but what better to chase someone with) because I am denying the existence of the infamous G-spot. I am not. I am only denying the anatomic location based on my study of anatomy in both text and cadaver alike. The text we studied in medical school for anatomy was called Netters. There are over 60 pages dedicated to the pelvis and perineum, 9 specifically for the nerves. It's not in there. I even pulled out my William's Gynecology, another reputable text that is comprehensive and factual. It's not there.

For those of you who KNOW that the G-spot exists, I'm happy for you. There are women who have never and will never experience this level of sensation, though. These women are not missing something that they are guaranteed anatomically. They just aren't. Sorry and RIP Dr. Gräfenberg. He was the dude who coined the term and theorized the location and function. (What was he doing in his spare time?) Even some sex therapists have been known to deny the existence in all women. The point is that women who have not experienced the G-spot should not consider themselves dysfunctional.

Wait, there is hope. Women are known for sexual individuality. What makes a woman's lady parts smile may not be limited to our textbooks or technical medical study. Don't give up on me yet. You own your sexuality! I am only trying to educate, enlighten, and occasionally entertain.

Annual Exams

Let's jump right in, or even better, scoot right on down.

"Doc, I'm told that I don't need a Pap test every year. Why should I see my Gyne every year?"

Reason #1 that you should see your Gyne every year...Because! Okay, that's not a reason. The first real reason is to check on how you are feeling and what has been going on with you in the last year. You may not know what's normal and what's not. Many women don't realize how many things happen to them in the course of a year and how those things can affect their overall health. I have had women forget that they had surgeries or new diagnoses until I ask questions about scars and new medications. Knowing how these events all work together is vital to keeping you safe. For example, a new diagnosis of high blood pressure, thyroid disease or seizure disorder may affect your birth control choice. A significant change in weight can sometimes point to a thyroid disorder. A change in your menstrual cycles can be normal or warrant further evaluation. These are just a few examples of relevant historical happenings.

Norms are also established at a yearly checkup. One woman's "normal" period flow may actually be excessive when put in perspective. I can look for signs of anemia, hormonal or structural abnormalities or reassure my patients when everything is actually normal. Unless you really spend time discussing your symptoms and comparing them to a group of truly normal friends and family, it may be hard to know if what you are experiencing is safe.

Reason #2 is to review your family history. It really matters! Family history can save you from experiencing the same fate. If a family member was diagnosed with colon or breast cancer, that information can change when your recommended screening mammograms and colonoscopies should begin—often sooner than average.

Let me take this moment to highlight the importance of asking your older family members about their medical problems and the importance of sharing your medical problems with younger family members. Many think that sharing medical problems like diabetes and cancer is "claiming it" or telling your "business." Instead, consider it a preview for things that you can see coming and prevent. Would you like to know when crossing the street that some cars and trucks may be coming around the corner beyond your line of sight? If you knew they were coming, would you cross a little more carefully? Would you look more closely? Would you behave a little more preventatively? If three of your family members developed diabetes, you may want to be screened earlier or be even more careful with your own weight and dietary choices. You may be able to either prevent the diagnosis altogether or at least catch it early before it causes too much harm.

Reason #3: To undergo a physical exam. I catch things that you may not. Blood pressure, weight, height (especially approaching or in menopause when osteoporosis can cause you to lose height), and physical exam findings can be vitally important to your health. I personally have diagnosed a number of thyroid masses and discovered breast lumps that were unknown to my patients. An enlarged uterus may point to fibroids. I want you to know all about your body, but it is my JOB to know it too.

Reason #4: To get a Pap test. Cervical cancer is one of the most preventable cancers that there is. In one of my first GynecobLogic.com blog posts, "What's Pap-pening," I explained what a Pap test is. If you have had a number of normal Pap tests, according to ASCCP guidelines* established in 2009 and reaffirmed in 2013, you may not need a Pap test every year. Since the Pap guidelines changed to less frequent screening, people often try to tell me that their "other doctor" told them they can have annual exams every 2-3 years. Well, change the name then. Call it your every-two-to-three-year exam. The only problem is that isn't a "thing." Screening guidelines for women still call for a yearly exam. During said visit, health history and family history are reviewed, a clinical breast exam is performed, a pelvic exam is performed to assess the size and contour of the uterus and ovaries, and testing for sexually transmitted infections is offered. Most insurance plans still cover these exams, as long as the topics covered are within the realm of prevention. I will also provide an order for a mammogram if you are 40 or older. I remind ladies of the need for a colonoscopy if they are 45 or older. If your last Pap was abnormal, you definitely need one in a year. Cervical cancer forms slowly, but I've seen substantial changes from one year to the next. I've seen women go from having a mildly abnormal Pap test to caught-it-in-the-nick-of-time almost-cancer. Don't play with your health. Get your Pap. If you are worried about the discomfort, check out my Speculum section.

* ASCCP is the American Society of Colposcopy and Cervical Pathology

Reason #5: To address any new medical concerns and

potentially be tested for sexually transmitted infections. Consider this a brief Explanation of Benefits—an EOB for you. The copayless, no out-of-pocket annual preventative check covered by your insurance policy covers basic yearly things like a discussion about updates in your medical history, a routine physical exam, and cervical cancer screening. If you have more medical issues that need to be addressed or tests that need to be performed, additional charges may be incurred that may require a copay, deductible or coinsurance payout. I don't make the rules, the insurance companies do.

Medicine is one of the few service industries that has a third party decide if and when you get paid for services rendered. The heyday of medicine is over. Docs are not rich beyond belief anymore. If I wanted to be rich, I would have tried to be the CEO of a private insurance company, not a doctor. Between abundant student loans and sparse reimbursements, a doc could EASILY live check to check. The point is not for anyone to cry for me. It is to understand that my ability to consult about multiple medical problems came at a price (and I am still paying richly). My time for consultation is not going to be free. If a business hired a consultant to fix problems on multiple levels of administration, they would bill and expect to receive payment for the services rendered and time spent tackling EACH issue. Medicine is no different. The struggle is real.

So, to answer the question, what is an annual exam and how frequently should it be done? It is a verbal and physical exam, and it should be done annually. Just because you may not need a yearly Pap, that doesn't exempt you as a woman from seeing your gynecologist annually. When I wrote about this in the blog, I included multiple pictures of perennial flowers. What can I say? They come back every year (rimshot, thank you, thank you).

B.

Bacterial Vaginosis
See Discharge. Follow your nose. #toofar?

Bartholin Cysts

A Bartholin gland cyst is a mucous filled collection that occurs within the vagina. The Bartholin glands (or greater vestibular glands) are located on either side of the opening of the vagina and are responsible for lubricating the vagina. If these glands, which are normally pea-sized, become blocked, they will fill and enlarge. The enlargement alone can cause asymmetry of the vulva, but if they become infected, they can be extremely painful. About 2% of women in their 20s will expect to have a Bartholin gland cyst at some point in their lives. The older women get, the less likely they are to develop Bartholin gland cysts or abscesses. Interestingly, Bartholin glands cysts in older women, especially recurrent ones, can be more concerning for cancer or precancerous potential. Removal is often the best solution in the older crowd.

Treatment of Bartholin gland cysts and abscesses vary. I have taken care of some women with asymptomatic cysts that were only mildly enlarged, stable in size, and not physically bothersome. To those women I say, "If it doesn't bother you, it doesn't bother me." For those with a larger and more annoying cyst, in its early stages, the cyst can be commonly managed with warm compresses and warm baths twice daily. If that doesn't help, a doctor may need to incise (cut) and drain the cyst or abscess. A recurrent or resistant cyst may need a catheter to be placed and left in the cyst. This is called a Word catheter. This allows the opening of the cyst to remain open long enough for the fluid within the cyst to not re-accumulate and gives it an opportunity for the cyst to heal. If none of that works, surgery may become necessary. The operation can either entail removing the gland completely or opening the cyst and essentially sewing it opened, a technique called Marsupialization. If you have never had a Bartholin gland cyst or abscess, be grateful. They hurt and are very disruptive to women's lives. They suck!

Birth Control

See Contraceptives.

Bloating

Stop everything. You have ovarian cancer. Okay, no you don't. Ovarian cancer is a very scary and sad disease. I only make light of it in this moment because so many women think that they have it; however, statistically, it is very uncommon. 2017 cancer statistics are as follows:

•   Ovarian cancer ranks fifth in cancer deaths among women, accounting for more deaths than any other cancer of the female reproductive system.

•   A woman's risk of getting ovarian cancer during her lifetime is about 1 in 75.

•   The average woman's chance of dying from it is about 1 in 100.

Unlike some other cancers, ovarian cancer is a very hard disease to diagnose. Other diseases often show you signs when they are present. Breast cancer often presents with a mass one can feel, or an abnormal finding on a routine mammogram. Skin cancer starts as an abnormal mole or lesion. Ovarian cancer, on the other hand, often has no symptoms at all until a woman is in advanced stages. There are also no routine screening tests for ovarian cancer. Late stage disease can make a woman feel fatigued, lose her appetite and feel bloated. These symptoms are non-specific, meaning they can be signs of anything. Who doesn't feel bloated at random times or around our menstrual cycle? See "O" for more ovarian cancer facts, but for now, consider periodic bloating a part of life. If coupled with other symptoms that concern you, definitely see your doctor.

My husband, gastroenterologist Dr. Ed McDonald IV, has a blog called The Doc's Kitchen (thedocskitchen.com) where he wrote an article all about the bloating as it relates to digestion. Check that out.

Body Blues

By definition, body blues is a type of depression. I thought that I had coined the term because I was thinking about how a person can be sad or depressed by the physical appearance of their body. I see women who try to get "thicker" with various types of implants or try to have thinner waists to be more physically attractive to potential partners. As a result of this desire, some women feel sad or depressed about their bodies. I am intrigued with this idea because we do laser body sculpting in our office. Part of my professional practice is to contour women's bodies so they feel better in their own skin. As a person who has used the laser myself (hey, I have three kids and HAD a belly to show for it), I can appreciate a woman's desire to change her physique without feeling bad about herself. Being proud within and still desiring a physical change in appearance are not mutually exclusive. It is okay for the two to coexist. Plenty of people with tremendously high self-esteem still go to the gym and wear nice clothes. I embrace the amazing parts of myself and am not ashamed to modify other parts. There are extremes, though, like the person who alters their appearance to the extent that they look completely different (R.I.P. Michael Jackson). It's their Bobby Brown Prerogative to "do what they want to do" to their face or body, but their self-love status could be called into question when extreme alterations are pursued.

My research of the lay term Body Blues did yield an actual definition, which was not the same as my made up one. Essentially it is a nickname for depression. Since the "D" section in this book has so many categories, let's tackle depression right here and now. The clinical diagnosis of depression usually means spending over 50% of the time feeling at least three of the following:

- Eating too much and gaining weight
- Lack of energy
- Irritability or tension
- Difficulty concentrating
- Sleep problems
- Daytime drowsiness
- Decreased interest in sex
- Mild anxiety
- Mild depression
- Heightened sensitivity to rejection or criticism

Apparently, I have had depression since I was born. Just kidding. I have had many of the fatigue-related symptoms since medical school, though. I want to take a nap right now because I'm at the hospital at midnight. For the record, I am not depressed now, but I definitely have been at different stages in my life. One of those stages was after the birth of my first son. I had an atypical manifestation.

My postpartum depression showed up as anger. I was pissed off, like, most of the time. I loved my little nugget, but breastfeeding and pumping did not evoke good feelings (no euphoria over here), eating was a chore, and my husband could do no right. He used to sit on the edge of the bed in the morning to put on his socks, and I would be boiling inside because it would make the mattress bounce just enough to wake me up. It was a small thing, especially since he was actually getting up to go to work and I was not, but I used to overflow with fury inside. I even tried to get rid of our dog in that timeframe because he was having accidents on the floor after we brought the baby home, maybe as a sign of rebellion against the new baby. I used to think "If you are trying to get me to choose between you and the baby, you won't win."

In my defense, if a grown man walked into your house and dropped a deuce on your floor, you would not let that man live with you. Our dog weighs about 130 pounds. That grown-up deuce almost lost his South Side Chicago residence.

The purpose of this diatribe (a forceful and bitter, verbal attack against someone or something) against myself is to highlight the fact that anyone can fall victim to mental health issues, whether temporarily or long term. I am a person who believes in getting help, whether with counseling or sometimes, even medication. If Molly on HBO's Insecure can go to "therapy," anyone can.

Breastfeeding

As a practicing OB/GYN and mother of three, breastfeeding is a topic that comes up in my conversations practically every day. This food source is truly "liquid gold," offering growing babies nutrition, protection and long-lasting health benefits. It's also advantageous for women. Breastfeeding women can experience faster weight loss, lower rates of postpartum depression and a stronger bond between mother and child.

Mothers labor to get their babies here, but breastfeeding is truly another labor of love. Though often challenging initially, it is worth every drop babies get. Here are 5 tips to help you successfully accomplish this goal:

1.   Provide yourself with the proper fuel. If you hope to produce a food source for another human being, you should take in the proper building blocks to create it. Continue taking prenatal vitamins (or postnatal vitamins if you prefer. They're essentially the same) and drink water frequently, even when you aren't thirsty. Eat nutritious foods: lean meats, beans, whole grains, well-washed or organic fruits and vegetables and dairy. Also, avoid excessive sugar.

2.   Don't get discouraged. Breastmilk can take up to five days

to come in for first-time mothers. Until then, the baby will be getting colostrum, a valuable nutritional source with antibodies for fighting infection. If you squeeze your nipple, you should be able to see the little clear or yellowish droplets form. Remember, newborns survived those first few days of life long before formula existed. Supply depends on demand. Let your baby nurse on demand. Your pediatrician will use your baby's weight and wet diaper count to ensure that the baby is getting enough food. If they recommend supplementation, listen. All women and all breasts are not created equally. Your baby's well-being is paramount.

3.   Those who can, do; those who can't, pump. Not every baby will latch onto the breast, even after using multiple techniques. Using a breast pump on each breast for at least 15 minutes every 2-3 hours will usually express enough milk to supply a newborn's needs. Working moms can breastfeed too. Having a breast pump can allow you the ability to nurse at home and pump at work. If your production is not enough to supply the baby's needs, something is better than nothing. Give your baby breastmilk in addition to formula. Your baby won't know the difference but will reap the benefits.

4.   Trouble doesn't last always. Breastfeeding is often uncomfortable in the beginning. This discomfort should get better. If it doesn't, seek help from a lactation consultant or your doctor. Clogged milk ducts, mastitis and engorgement can cause severe pain. Massage, warm compresses and expressing milk every 1.5 to 2 hours when painful nodules arise can help to prevent the development of infection.

5.   Know when enough is enough. If you have tried every trick in the book and are still unable to breastfeed, sometimes the healthiest thing for a mother's emotional well-being is to accept this reality and let it go. As valuable as breastmilk is, it is not worth the negative effects on one's psyche when it just doesn't work out.

Breast Health

Monthly self-breast exams are still my recommendation. The American College of Obstetrics and Gynecology (ACOG) previously recommended monthly self-breast exams and yearly clinical breast exams performed by a doctor. The recommendations also included yearly screening mammograms to begin at age 40 or 10 years earlier than your closest relative at their age of breast cancer diagnosis. Now the guidelines are a little, well... a little lumpy. #cantstopwontstop

Monthly self-breast exams are no longer recommended across the board based on the evidence, and some research discourages them because of the likelihood of a woman finding a mass or lump that is benign (not cancerous), resulting in a lot of follow up testing, biopsies and mental anguish. My non-evidence based take on it is that YOU should make the choice. Only about 20% of lumps detected on self-exam will be cancer. The other 80% can cause anxiety if you let them, but just don't freak out. If you don't check, you have to be okay with not finding anything, even if there is a cancer present. Following this logic, not checking at all is better than possibly finding a cancer that could be treated and possibly save your life. But what about the stats that say anywhere between 20-40% of breast cancers are detected by self-exam? I don't know about you, but I don't like to keep my head in the sand (and not just because of my hair).

Mammograms are recommended starting at age 50 or age 45 or age 40, depending on which guidelines you check. The frequency and timing (yearly vs. every two years) depend on a woman's personal and family history. Together, my patient and I can go through pros and cons and decide which timing seems most reasonable. The cons are similar to those for self-breast exams. For one, a large number of suspicious findings will be benign. Also, cancers that develop earlier in age are more likely to be aggressive, so early detection may not decrease mortality (the likelihood of death). Ultimately, then, you could say that how often you screen depends on how much information you want to know. Would you feel better knowing that your breasts are cancer free, even if it means going back for more testing, or would you rather assume they are cancer free and not get checked, even if there is a small chance that something abnormal is there? As for me, I want to know, even if that means running more tests.

ACOG provides much of the evidence and recommendations that guide our practice of medicine. Let's stop for a second and examine this term "evidence" as in "evidence-based medicine". The NIH defines this term as the conscientious, explicit, judicious and reasonable use of modern, best evidence in making decisions about the care of individual patients. Evidence-based medicine integrates clinical experience and patient values with the best available research information. I had to highlight that definition early in this book because, with the help of Google and Facebook Mom's groups (no one specific #nooffense), a single post or article can feel like it represents everyone. Keep in mind, people often post or write about experiences when they are different or unique. The other 99% of people who had normal or typical or average experiences don't blog or take an hour or more out of their lives to write about them. Individual experiences aren't evidence. I digress. #whyiwrite

Monthly self-breast exams help women to find breast changes or abnormalities sooner than they would normally be found by a yearly gynecologic exam. I see you once a year. You see yourself every day. To try to justify not doing self-exams, women often tell me one of two things: Either they don't know how to do these exams or they don't know what is normal vs. abnormal. What I tell those women is "Friend, get up in there! They're yours, right?"

How to do a self-breast exam?

Firmly but comfortably press through the entire breast in a systematic way to be sure to feel all breast tissue. Don't leave out the area under the nipple or under the armpit because breast tissue extends into those areas. The question of how one knows what is abnormal can be answered by knowing what is normal. You don't have to be a breast expert, but you should be your own breast expert. Do these exams after your period or, if you don't have monthly periods because of your birth control type, do them around the same time every month. If you know your breasts well—the densities, the texture, etc.—then you will be the first to know if something changes or a new nodule or frozen pea pops up.

The term "frozen pea" is used commonly in the medical community to refer to a breast lump that doesn't move when you push on it. It can be the size of a pea, and it feels non-mobile and hard in the breast. That type of lump is more concerning than the mobile lump that is easily pushed around. A patient recently told me that her breast doctor referred to these easily moveable lumps as "breast mice." Breast Mice? That is a TERRIBLE name for anything within a woman's body. Maybe I take this one so personally because I have lived in a domicile (a few domiciles) with mice in the past. The last thing I want to think about is having one inside my breast. Consider this my own attempt to change that term to one more pleasing to my ear: "non-cancerous breast nodules commonly feel like fruit in breast Jello." No? Well, as I am typing this I immediately thought of Bill Cosby. So much for that attempt. I'll think of something better than "breast mice."

What if you find something abnormal in the breast? Rruht rroh (insert Scooby-Doo voice). What if you have a breast pain, a lump or a bump, or discharge coming from the nipple. There are many breast changes that can occur and some are scarier than others. Dense or lumpy areas that arise just before the period and go away shortly thereafter are far less concerning than a new firm lump that is painless and doesn't move well. A small, rock-like structure in the breast that is not freely mobile may be that way because the tissue around it is scarred. Cancer causes scarring. Any breast finding that is new or not quickly resolving warrants some attention. That attention could mean making a mental note to check on it daily or every other day until your period comes to see if it goes away. Or that attention could mean that you call your gynecologist and schedule an appointment to have it checked out.

When I evaluate someone for breast concerns, I will typically listen to the history of its onset, do a physical examination, and give my best opinion and recommendations about their signs and symptoms. Those recommendations may be to wait a little while for it to resolve, or it may be to get a mammogram or an ultrasound. For my ladies who want further imaging when I don't recommend it, I tell them that I will order the evaluation if their peace of mind is at stake.

Some doctors may take issue with this approach. They may think that since we go to school for half of our lives, we should be trusted to make the right decisions for diagnosis and treatment of our patients. We should. I too believe that. The flaw in adhering to that philosophy, without exception, is that we are all adults and can make our own decisions in life. This is the entire concept of informed consent. I present you with your options, the pros and cons of each option, and my recommendations. You can then make your own decision. If you won't be able to sleep at night until that breast ultrasound report says benign, who am I to deny that piece of mind, even if I think that it is unnecessary. At the end of the day, it is your body and I am here to help you stay safe both mentally and physically. Also, I am not flawless. Sometimes a woman's intuition can trump a doctor's knowledge.

If you suspect a new breast lump, as with any health concern, don't ignore it. Ignoring the symptoms won't make them go away. Either time will pass and it will get better, or time will pass and the symptoms will get worse. You would hate to know that if you have acted sooner, you may have improved your health or even saved your own life.

Here is what the American Cancer Society has to say about prevention of breast cancer:

1. Because obesity and excess weight increase the risk of developing breast cancer, the American Cancer Society recommends that women maintain a healthy weight throughout their life. Losing even a small amount of weight has health benefits and is a good place to start.

2. Growing evidence suggests that women who get regular physical activity have a 10%-25% lower risk of breast cancer compared to women who get no exercise. Doing even a little physical activity beyond your regular daily routine can have many health benefits.

3. Many studies have confirmed that drinking alcohol increases the risk of breast cancer in women by about 7% to 10% for each drink per day. For women who drink alcohol, the American Cancer Society recommends they limit themselves to no more than 1 drink per day.

4. There is some scientific evidence that smoking increases the risk of breast cancer slightly, especially among heavy, long-term smokers and women who begin smoking before their first pregnancy. A recent study by American Cancer Society researchers found that women who begin smoking before they give birth to their first child had a 21% higher risk of breast cancer than women who never smoked. Quitting has numerous health benefits.

5. To find breast cancer early, when treatments are more likely to be successful, the American Cancer Society recommends women should begin having yearly mammograms by age 45 and can change to having mammograms every other year beginning at age 55. Women should have the choice to start screening with yearly mammograms as early as age 40 if they want to.

For all my sisters in the struggle, you think I've forgotten about you (yes, I'm quoting/stealing from "I've Been Looking for You" by Kirk Franklin). I haven't. The only thing I will add, that is specific to African American women, is that breast cancer occurs in African American women at a slightly lower rate than Caucasian women, but we are significantly more likely to die from the disease than Caucasian women—42% more likely to be exact. This is partly because the disease onset is earlier and thus not detected as soon, and it is often more aggressive. This is even more of a reason to do self-exams, to see your doctor yearly, and to be aware of your family history and discuss it with your doctor.

Bump

Looking for information about a bump on your lady parts? Go to the Lesion section for this topic.

C.

Cancer

I was in medical school before I really understood what cancer was, so I thought it deserved a section. Plus practically everyone who I call and tell about their abnormal Pap test thinks they have cervical cancer until they are talked off of the ledge.

Cancer is not an alien beast that finds its way into your body. Cancer, generally speaking, is caused by rogue cells of your own body. Our whole body is composed of cells, tiny building blocks with specific functions that work together. When a few cells decide to do their own thing, it is like a mutiny. I recently watched Guardians of the Galaxy 2. *Spoiler alert*. When Yondu's crew was overthrown by Taserface, they killed all of the loyal crewmates by tossing them off of the ship into the vacuum of space. Taserface was like a cancer, turning the formerly good crewmates against Yondu.

If we keep with the cancer analogy, the newly corrupted crew members would have started multiplying and forming new corrupt crew members like that agent in the black suit with the earpiece in the Matrix #The90s. Eventually, those crew members would multiply beyond capacity, use up all of the resources, food and water on the ship, and everyone would die. That's cancer. The way that chemotherapy works to stop it is that it targets the cells that replicate quickly. Cells that rapidly divide and multiply use certain building blocks that chemotherapy and radiation can target and attack. Hair follicles also have rapidly dividing cells, which is why people lose their hair during chemotherapy.

There is also a component of cancer that results from a deficiency in eliminating malfunctioning cells. Let me try that again. When cells don't function well, there are proteins that are supposed to cause those cells to die. It's like a gardener who pulls up weeds and prunes rogue branches on bushes. If the gardener isn't doing a good job, parasitic weeds can overgrow and overtake the whole garden. Good luck to your delicate herb garden when big chunky weeds go unchecked. The weed analogy gives the visual, but just to reiterate, the cancer cells are not foreign. They are cells that were at one point functioning normally in your body which just decided for one reason or another to malfunction.

Malfunctioning cells can be caused by infection (HPV for example), smoking (it's not just the cause of lung cancer), poor diet (processed foods are just one culprit), or plain old family history. If a close family member got colon cancer before the age of 50, or even polyps, your screening colonoscopies may need to start at age 40 or younger. You may have some genes that make your gardeners stop working, or your Taserface is super bold.

A healthy diet rich in antioxidants can also help to knock out bad cells and bad genes like a good dodgeball player will knock out the weaklings first. Green leafy veggies and omega-3 fatty acids found in many types of fish are just two dietary choices that can decrease your cancer risk. Processed foods are also a rising cause of cancer formation. More on that from Dr. Ed McDonald over at thedocskitchen.com. #shamelessplug #itsgoodstuff

The most common cancers:
For Women:
1. Breast cancer
2. Lung cancer
3. Colorectal cancer
4. Uterine cancer

For Men:
1. Prostate cancer
2. Lung cancer
3. Colorectal cancer
The list of the most common cancer DEATHS in the US, not

considering ethnicity are:
1. Lung and bronchial cancer
2. Colon and rectal cancer
3. Breast cancer
4. Pancreatic cancer
5. Prostate cancer
6. Leukemia
7. Non-Hodgkin lymphoma
8. Liver and intrahepatic bile duct cancer

Cancer screening is meant to catch signs of cancer when it is early and small enough to treat. Personally, I plan on having yearly mammograms starting at age 40 and screening colonoscopies starting at age 45, unless my personal or family history suggests otherwise. And I'll never smoke because that increases the chance of contracting and dying from every cancer that exists.

Candidiasis

Also known as yeast. My arch nemesis. The bane of my existence. Is my disdain for this itchy, irritating, spontaneous infection a dead giveaway to my own T.M.I.? Maybe. I wrote a poem about how much I can't stand yeast. I didn't actually, but there is definitely a song in my heart about it. Wait for it.

My father nicknamed me Sweets as a child. He called me that because of my affinity for all things sugary and sweet. Could my "candy girl" beginnings be a reason for the turmoil that my body has endured throughout the years? Sidebar—I can only hope that my dad is not reading this because somehow my dad knowing about my trials and tribulations with this pesky infection is more embarrassing than all of my readers (thanks to you all) knowing about it. Funny. Any-who, candidiasis, or yeast, can be extremely bothersome and sometimes difficult to rid the body of. Those of you who have never had one, consider yourselves very, very lucky. Those who have, the itching, irritation and sometimes even pain of excessive inflammation can be distracting and difficult to manage. I have coined the term "double-dutch vagina" for my ladies who are so frequently graced with yeast or bacterial infections, they have to catch the vagina at the perfect time for intimate moments. Imagine trying to hurry up and let the bedroom good times roll before the vagina betrays you again. Yeast sucks. See Discharge for more about bacterial vaginitis and other annoying vaginal infections.

The diagnosis of yeast isn't always as intuitive as you would think. My mantra is "everything that itches isn't yeast." Some stats say that as many as three out of four women who think they have a yeast infection are wrong. Baseline symptoms of yeast include itching/irritation and discharge, though some women with yeast infections don't have discharge. Take-home message: If you try to treat suspected yeast without improvement, go see your doctor.

Cesarean Section

Commonly known as C-section, cesarean delivery is the method of delivering a baby through the abdomen rather than through the vagina. A horizontal (bikini cut), or sometimes vertical incision is made on the abdomen and the baby is delivered through it. The muscles of the abdomen are separated but rarely cut. The bowels and bladder are usually either already out of the vicinity or are pushed out of the way to accomplish this delivery without complications. The more abdominal surgeries a woman has had, such as C-sections and myomectomies, the more likely there is to be a complication. Injury to the bowel, bladder, ureters, and other vessels and organs becomes more likely because scar tissue is there to distort the normal anatomy.

Some people want C-sections because of the desire to preserve the contour of the vagina or to avoid the challenges in bladder control that can arise after a vaginal delivery. Some need a cesarean because the baby is not head down, the baby is extremely large, or there are multiple babies that make the delivery more dangerous through the vagina. Some don't find out until they are in labor that their baby is unable to tolerate labor, or that their uterus is not contracting well enough to get them to 10 centimeters dilation, or that their cervix is unwilling to comply and dilate, or that their baby won't fit through their pelvis despite pushing or attempted vacuum or forceps delivery.

Some examples of women who should have a C-section are women whose first vaginal delivery resulted in a shoulder dystocia, which is when the baby gets stuck coming out. Because there can be a lack of oxygen while the baby is stuck, and because shoulder dystocias often happen with subsequent deliveries, the risks of a C-section are way less than the complications that can result if a baby has a severe dystocia. Also, a woman who had an extensive tear through the vagina and rectum with her first delivery (a 4th-degree tear) should be offered a C-section with the second. Scar tissue is weak, so the chance of having a second 4th-degree laceration is high. Healing becomes more challenging, and if you don't heal well from that type of tear, you risk fecal or flatus incontinence—losing stool or gas without control. Not cool dude. C-section me.

Factors that can increase your chances of needing a C-section are being overweight or obese, having diabetes, or being over 35 at the time of delivery, among others. Some of these things you can't control, but starting off at a healthy weight can make a difference.

So what happens if you have a C-section for the first delivery? Can you try to deliver vaginally next time? Sure. That is called a VTOL or TOLAC. VTOL stands for vaginal trial of labor. TOLAC stands for trial of labor after cesarean. Both are possible after one cesarean section, and in some cases, after two cesarean deliveries. Two things that are important to know about VTOL/TOLACs are that the reason for the first delivery matters and the risk of uterine rupture should always be clear to all parties. A person who had a C-section because the baby was breech (feet down rather than head down) or didn't tolerate labor is a better candidate to attempt a VTOL than someone who had a labor that never got to 10 centimeters of dilation despite adequate effort or someone who couldn't push a baby out despite trying. There is a calculator that we use from MFMU.com, which is a source created by the high-risk obstetricians. It allows a clinician to plug in demographic and medical history information to give a percentage success rate. If the calculator says that a woman's chance of having a successful VBAC is at least 60% or greater, we as OB/GYNs should offer this to her. If the percent is lower or the last C-section was less than 18 months from the last delivery to anticipated delivery, a scheduled C-section is preferred.

What is all the ruckus about VTOL being dangerous? Well, the concern is uterine rupture. As I mentioned, with severe vaginal lacerations, scars are weak. Where the uterus was cut previously during a C-section, the muscle is not as strong as the rest of the uterus. That means when the uterus contracts and puts strain on the previously cut area, that area is at risk for opening. That risk is about 1%, without the aid of augmentation like Pitocin or misoprostol. With augmentation, the risk goes up. One percent is a very low risk, which is why so many clinicians do VTOLs. Even though complications arise infrequently, when they do occur, they can be devastating. Mom's and baby's lives are both at risk, and long-term medical problems are not uncommon. Extensive counseling and risk assessment are key.

How many C-sections can a woman have? As many as she wants, but with each one, especially after having had three, the risk of the placenta abnormally adhering to the uterus increases. This is called a placenta accreta, and it can lead to an increased risk for hemorrhage, hysterectomy during delivery, and loss of life. I caution ladies about having more than three C-sections. To reiterate, I'm not saying that a person can't have ten children via C-section if they want to. I can't make decisions about your child count, but the safety risks are real.

The bottom line is that if you need to have C-section, you need it. If your doc's C-section rate is dramatically above 30%, which is the national average, you may need to discuss why and reconsider your choice of provider. I remember a wise doc I trained under who used to say that his C-section rate was 100% when it had to be. He made no apologies for keeping mom and baby safe. I love a vaginal delivery like the next doc, but I don't apologize for getting mom and baby through the delivery process unscathed, even if that means bright lights and cold steel. Any mother would prefer a scar at her bikini line over an oxygen-deprived baby through her vagina ANY DAY.

Sidebar about the incontinence (bladder leakage) concerns— studies show that women can still have bladder control issues after just carrying a baby, regardless of how the baby comes out. A C-section to avoid possible incontinence in the future may not be worth it.

Regarding pregnancies with multiple children, like twins or triplets, they can sometimes come out vaginally. It depends on how far along they are based on the due date, and how they are positioned. If the first twin is head down and bigger than the second one, one can sometimes try to deliver them vaginally, but there is always a chance that after the first comes out, the second can have a complication that requires an emergent C-section. All parties have to be aware of that possibility before the delivery is attempted.

At the end of the day, if you don't want any chance of having a C-section, don't get pregnant. If you find yourself pregnant, resolve early in the pregnancy that 1 in 3 women in the US have a cesarean delivery. You want a safe and healthy baby, right? There are two ways to get you and baby across that finish line. Wrap your head around it. More on this subject in the Pregnancy and Labor sections.

Cervix

The cervix is essentially the opening to the uterus. It is also the conduit for pregnancy and, possibly, infection. It is the place where Pap tests are performed to screen for pre-cancer and cancer of the cervix. See the Anatomy section for more about the cervix location and function. See Human Papillomavirus and Pap sections for additional information.

Circumcision

In the state where I practice, Illinois, the OB/GYNs perform circumcisions on baby boys. This is in contrast to places where a pediatrician is responsible for surgery on this very personal organ. I often get asked, "Why would an obstetrician, who otherwise is only usually responsible for babies while their umbilical cord is attached to the uterus, now be in charge of removal of the foreskin from a baby's penis?" The answer is because we are the surgeons. We do C-sections and hysterectomies. I also remove skin tags, perform revision of the external vagina, known as labioplasty, etc. When was the last time you saw a pediatrician wielding a scalpel?

Do I recommend circumcisions? No. Do I discourage women or men from having their baby boys circumcised? No. Are my boys circumcised? None of your beeswax. The decision to circumcise in the US is mostly cultural and cosmetic. The American Pediatric Association does not recommend that all boys get circumcised. Informed consent is a practice in medicine where you make sure that a person understands the risks, benefits and alternatives so they can make an informed decision. The risks of circumcision are bleeding, infection and damage to the penis. These risks are extremely low and the device that I use protects the penis itself and only exposes the foreskin. This makes causing any harm to the penis extremely unlikely.

A benefit of performing this procedure when a baby is only a day or two old, rather than later in life, is that the anesthesia requirement is minimal. I use lidocaine to numb the area in similar fashion to a dentist using lidocaine to numb the mouth during dental work. It takes about one week to heal with little to no perceived discomfort to the baby. Feed and swaddle a baby, and he'll do just fine. Diaper changes can sometimes be a time when boys seem to show a little more animosity toward their parents in the first days after circumcision, but after about one week, it is healed.

In a child dealing with recurrent urinary tract infections or constriction of the foreskin, known as priapism, circumcision may be recommended and necessary at some point. Situations like those are uncommon.

In adults, data shows less STD transmission in circumcised men. The reason for this is simple: surface area. Uncircumcised men have a bigger proverbial net to catch cooties. That doesn't mean that they absolutely will, though. A common myth is that circumcised penises are cleaner. I have had women blame their recurrent yeast or other vaginitis on their uncircumcised partner. First of all, many of these ladies need to carry and use a condom. STD transmission is not intentional. Someone can care for you, even love you, but please don't mistake serial monogamy for a negative STD test. We'll get more into STDs in later chapters, but the point is that while uncircumcised men carry a slightly higher risk of infection transmission, that doesn't mean that an original, unrevised penis is "dirty". Couples who I have cared for who have decided not to circumcise their babies often do so because the father is not circumcised. This sounds like TMI, but the subject often comes up while discussing how to care for an uncircumcised penis. The dads always say that it isn't hard to care for and they will teach their sons what they need to know. That learning curve is a little different if the parents are trying to break the circumcision cycle. Your pediatrician can aid in counseling and guidance. You can't exactly YouTube care of an uncircumcised penis. Well, maybe you can, but you probably shouldn't. Ask someone who knows.

Cold Sores

So innocent, so common, so HERPES. This may come as a surprise to some but not to others. There is more extensive information about Herpes Simplex Virus, or HSV, presented in the STD section of this book, but here is the quick and dirty on cold sores (#punlife.) There are 2 different types of Herpes Simplex Virus, Type 1 and Type 2. Type 1 is commonly found in the oral region and presents as "fever blisters", or painful red blisters on the lips or nose. They are found specifically on keratinized skin, or the skin found on the outside of the body, rather than the moist mucosa of the inner mouth. Painful lesions on the inside of the mouth are commonly canker sores, among other possibilities.

An uncommonly known fact is that HSV Type 2 can also be present orally, though it is the type of HSV most commonly found genitally. Conversely, HSV-1 can be found genitally even though it is usually oral. I have definitely seen patients diagnosed with vulvovaginal herpes after only oral sex and with cultures that prove the traditionally oral type of the virus. Statistically, per the NIH (the National Institute of Health), the prevalence of HSV-1 in the population is 65%. Globally, it is theorized that 90% of people have been exposed to HSV-1, HSV-2 or both. More on HSV-2 in the section entitled Questions.

What are cold sore take-home points?

1. It's all Herpes, no matter how you slice it.

2. It is very contagious. So many children have "fever blisters" because of some adult's innocent displays of affection. If you have a lesion or have recently had one, don't kiss your kids on the face, let alone on the lips. No judgment, but I didn't grow up in a lip-kissing household anyway.

3. No one is safe unless you restrict contact. Obviously, if someone has active lesions, that is a given, but even if a person is asymptomatic, they could still have AND SPREAD the virus. This is called asymptomatic shedding. To be put another way, a person who carries the virus may or may not know they carry the virus and may be able to spread the virus to another person without showing any signs of being contagious. This is why so many people have the virus. It is so sneaky, and once you have it, you can never completely rid your body of it.

The good news is that despite those troubling facts, it is a very benign virus in that it does not cause significant illness in most cases. Recurrences are a nuisance more than anything, and a strong immune system, coupled with the aid of medications when necessary, can keep it at bay. Stay tuned for more in the STD section of this book.

Colposcopy

This is the procedure used to evaluate a cervix after an abnormal Pap result. The Pap test uses a brush to sweep the cervix and collect cells randomly. If any of those cells are found to be abnormal, the colposcopy is performed to look more closely. Imagine that you swept your floor with a Roomba (I wish. I want one…), and when you emptied it, you saw ants or termites. You would then go back around your house and try to find where they were and see how bad the infestation is. That is what a colposcopy does. I use a microscope of sorts, a Colposcope to be exact, and I look closely at the whole cervix. I use a solution and a special light that makes abnormalities easier to see. If I see anything abnormal, I take a biopsy of that area and send it to my pathologist who will tell me what the damage is. If changes on the cervix are mildly abnormal, we can watch and wait and check again next year with a Pap. If they are severely abnormal, a part of the cervix may need to be removed. More on that in the Pap section.

Contraceptives

Before diving into this topic, there is a basic principle that we must address:

Vagina + Penile Sex in Man + Woman = Egg + Sperm = Baby.

I have to break down the basics because I often hear statements like this:

"I only did it once."

"We weren't trying."

"How did this happen?"

I ask every patient if they are sexually active. If they say, "Yes," then I ask if they are using condoms or any other form of birth control. If they say, "No," then I say, "Do you want to get pregnant?" The question is not a sarcastic one, nor is it meant to embarrass the patient. The answer is almost always an emphatic, "NO."

Then the pause… because if you aren't trying to get

pregnant, what are you doing to prevent it? When I hear, "Well, I don't have sex that much," I can't help but think, do you think you only produce a baby after having a certain amount of sex? Sure couples can try for a long time to get pregnant, but it only takes one time to actually conceive. If you remember the movie, Look Who's Talking, the classic '80s movie with John Travolta and Kirstie (I thought her name was Kristie for the longest) Alley, the sperm swims and swims and gains admission to the egg to make the hilarious talking baby who we all fell in love with. That conception scene was amazing, timeless, and still available for viewing on YouTube. Did you know Bruce Willis was the voice of Mikey? Summary of this point: If you aren't preventing pregnancy, you ARE "trying." Oh and the pull-out method doesn't count. I have a music video called "My Boo" on dreverywoman.com and YouTube about this topic. It features that '90s song from the running man challenge. Go ahead, you are excused. Come back when you are done. Keyword: dreverywoman.

On average, not adjusting for age or risk factors, after one year of unprotected intercourse, 86 out of 100 women will get pregnant. Pull-out decreases chances of conception, but enough semen is released prior to ejaculation to leave a substantial chance of conceiving. To be specific, in one year of regular unprotected sex using the pull-out method, 22 women out of 100 will be pregnant. The Rhythm method will leave 24 out of 100 women pregnant, and a startling 18 women will be pregnant who use the traditional male condom (sorry rubbers). Part of that risk comes from improper or inconsistent use, while part of it comes from failure of the method itself (a hole in the condom for example). I still believe wholeheartedly in condoms for reducing STD transmission. Condoms are not perfect, but apart from abstinence, they are better than nothing. The sole use of condoms is not the best pregnancy prevention, though. The most comprehensive and accurate contraceptive statistics can be found on the Center for Disease Control (CDC) website. My favorite options include implants and IUDs. Less than 1 pregnancy per 100 women in one year sounds like a winner to me. These methods aren't for everyone, but they will bring your "surprise pregnancy" chances down substantially.

Anyway, if you don't want to get pregnant, but you do want to have sex, birth control is a must-have EVERY TIME. The only absolute 100% effective form of contraception is abstinence, which

I believe in, support, and practiced myself in my pre-marital days, (TMI). Now that I've made that statement, let's tackle types of contraception: barrier, pill, patch, ring, shot, IUD, implant and permanent sterilization.

Barrier methods include condoms and diaphragms with spermicide. Yes, some women still use diaphragms. A diaphragm is fit to a woman's uniquely sized vagina by a gynecologist in the office and is then ordered at the pharmacy. Proper diaphragm use entails filling the rubber cup with spermicide and placing it in the vagina. A diaphragm can be inserted as many as six hours before intercourse and should stay in place for six hours after intercourse. The reason for this is that the spermicide-diaphragm combo has to remain in place long enough to kill the sperm and block passage to the uterus. If that isn't sexy enough for you, there are other options that can possibly do the trick.

There are different kinds of birth control pills. The term "the pill" can include combined estrogen-progesterone pills (COCs) or progesterone-only pills. Over the course of a year on a pill, 9 women out of 100 will become pregnant. COCs stop you from ovulating or releasing an egg, and they regulate the menstrual cycle. Estrogen-containing birth control needs to be used with caution in smokers and women over the age of 35, and shouldn't be used in women with certain types of migraines, cancer, or blood clotting disorders. Blood clotting disorders are not to be confused with blood clots that may come out of your body during a heavy period. The clotting disorders that are contraindicated with (shouldn't be used with) COCs or estrogen are the ones that develop deep clots within the veins of the legs or lungs. These blood clots can be life-threatening. Increased estrogen levels can make them more likely to form. Progesterone only pills, implants or IUDs, or even hormone-free IUDs may be options for women with clotting disorders. For the sake of perspective, the risk of developing a blood clot from birth control is about 4 in 10,000, or 0.04%. On an estrogen-containing birth control, the risk is about 10-14 in 10,000, or about 0.1%. In pregnancy, the risk is about 5 times that of the no birth control group (the NBCs as I just decided to call them), which is 0.2% (1 in 500). The risk is about 20 times higher in the postpartum period than the NBCs, or about 1% (1 in 100).

Permanent options like tubal ligation during C-section and laparoscopic tubal ligation are all effective methods of birth control.

You MUST be ABSOLUTELY SURE you don't want to have any, or any more, babies when you choose this method. There is no consistently successful reversal of a tubal ligation and the risks are not small when attempting to restore fertility. When I ask my patients if they want their tubes tied, say in the setting of a scheduled C-section, if they say, "I think I do," with the pensive, unsure emoji hovering over their head, I generally respond by saying, "You didn't say it right." You need to know that you know that you know that you don't want to have any more children EVER. If you aren't 100% certain, a LARC (long- acting REVERSIBLE contraceptive) can offer you the same effectiveness with the reversibility in case you really do change (or in my case, lose) your mind and want more children.

I know you didn't think I was going to make my way through the contraceptive topic without talking about vasectomy. Sure, the penis is not my organ of specialty, but a vasectomy is a very reasonable method of contraception. It is one of the least invasive methods of permanent contraception. You just need to make sure that the man goes for that confirmatory test ensuring no sperm remain in to ejaculate after the procedure. Initially, the situation is like that of pipes after you turn the water off. You have to get the remaining water out of the plumbing before you start disconnecting pipes. Tell him I said, "It's okay." Manly men get "snipped" too. He can crush a beer can on his forehead and go mow the lawn bare-chested after it's all done.

"How will birth control impact my long-term fertility?"
You shouldn't worry significantly about fertility after birth control, any more than you would worry about fertility not having been on birth control. The modifiable factor that matters most for fertility is not the length of time you have been on birth control. It is the age that you try to conceive. Fertility changes every year. There is not a magical change that occurs at the age of 35 as many women believe. Every year from when we start menstruating until we become menopausal, our fertility is decreasing and our risks of complications increase. This is a gradual change that becomes slightly more rapid at 32 and even 35, but a 22-year-old is more fertile than a 27-year-old, who is more fertile than a 32-year-old. While some women have menstrual cycle irregularities that may take a small amount of time to normalize after stopping birth control, some women get pregnant while on birth control, meaning there isn't a purge period that every

woman automatically needs in order to resume fertility.

The take-home point: Use whatever method suits you best for as long as you don't want to conceive, but never take fertility for granted because you don't know what hand you'll be dealt when you are "ready." Oh, and being 40-plus is NOT considered birth control. Surprise babies can occur all of the way up to menopause. The little miracles!

Birth control is not just for birth control anymore. Women use different methods to control bleeding and to regulate cycles, or sometimes to get rid of the period altogether. See M for more about menstrual cycles. My brain and my ovaries need a break after this chapter.

2
YOUNG ME WITH STETHOSCOPE DREAMS

Humble Chicago beginnings.

I am descended from greatness. My father is credited for bringing the Popeye's franchise to Chicago. Do you like your Chicago version of "Louisiana Fast?" Well, thank my daddy, William "Bill" Goodall, for those finger-lickin' goods. I am a first-generation Chicagoan. My father was born in Glen White, West Virginia, and my mother is from Louisville, Mississippi, not to be confused with Louisville, Kentucky. I also learned at an early age that Louisville, Mississippi is pronounced Lewis-ville, whereas that city in Kentucky is pronounced Lou-a-vul.

During my upbringing, my parents often shared stories of their childhood in the Jim Crow era. My dad and his brothers were chased on multiple occasions by young white boys throwing rocks at them because they were black. Their young formative years shaped how they viewed the world and our society. This translated into my childhood being full of cautions about subliminal AND overt racism. Racial innuendos were everywhere, from cartoons to toys. My mother and father were sure to keep our race-dar (get it? Instead of radar?) at highest sensitivity. I couldn't blame them for keeping their children on the alert for social injustices. They lived through some of the worst injustices since slavery. I would be lying if I didn't admit to believing that some of their sirens for racism were, in my opinion, hyper-examined pseudo-stereotypes. I did see some.

Racism is alive and well. That is a fact. If you doubted this truth during the Obama presidency (how could you have?), you certainly cannot deny it in the Trump Era.

Moving on, I have wanted to be a gynecologist since I was in pre-school. Slow down, you imaginative readers who are already questioning why a child would want to be an OB/GYN. The answer is much more innocent than you might think. I was a sucker for commercials then and now. There was this cool bath soap that I saw on TV and begged my mother to get. It came in what looked like a toothpaste tube, and it was both bright red and bright blue. In the commercials, happy, bubbly children drew fun pictures on their wash towel (before the days of widespread loufa usage) and wash their pictures into sudsy cleanliness. I was so excited to try it. After a few days of drawing blobs of not-cute pictures on my wash towel, I became increasingly irritated in the nether-region.

How this subject came up with my childhood best friend, I cannot recall. The part of the story that I do remember is that her mom was an OB/GYN, and she shared with me, in child speak, that some vaginas are more sensitive than others. Essentially, not everyone can handle exposure of her most sensitive areas to fragrant or colorful body products. When I sadly threw away that not-as-fun-as-I-thought-it-would-be body wash, my vagina stopped complaining.

How cool was it that Dr. My-Friend's-Mom (remember when you didn't know last names, but every grown-up was known as their-child's-name's Mom) knew with confidence what was wrong with me? It was clear to me that any person whose job and livelihood was to know everything she could know about the human body was someone I wanted to be like when I grew up. My body was a book that I could study and master, and with that masterful knowledge, I could help other women to be healthier and happier. The thought of that was amazing, even in my youth. Now on to my quest.

My parents bought me every supportive learning toy that I asked for. We had an IBM computer in the late '80s, complete with those large floppy disk drives. They found an academic computer program where you had to label the body parts and drag and drop them onto the proper anatomical locations of the human body. This is where I first learned to distinguish in the most rudimentary, low resolution, monochromatic form, the tibia from the fibula and the radius from the ulna. Those are the bones in the forearm and lower leg #fyi.

By far my favorite toy, academic or otherwise, was a plastic female figure called The Invisible Woman. If you are thinking of the superhero from The Fantastic Four, think again. It wasn't her. My IW (OB/GYNs love to abbreviate everything with acronyms) was a clear plastic shell of a woman which had the woman's complete set of organs and bones that came apart and could be put back together for 3D puzzle-like placement. The best part of her was that you could remove the abdominal plate and her small intestines, and replace that void with a pregnant uterus and another clear plastic pregnant shell that covered said uterus. Wait, it gets better. You could open the uterus like an Easter egg and A BABY WAS INSIDE. A head-down, 3rd-trimester baby! I was in the '80s version of Doc McStuffins heaven.

Doogie, or Doogina Howser I was not. I was not a child prodigy by any means. I went to a school full of geniuses where my level of intelligence was mediocre, or good at best. That bar was set HIGH. You don't believe me? I remember coming back to school from summer break one year in elementary school, and two of the kids had spent the entire summer trying to discover the next five digits of pi. You remember pi right? That geometric or trigonometric number that is defined to be the ratio of a circle's circumference to its diameter. The value of pi is slightly greater than three, or 3.14159… Did you know that pi has close to a million digits? So I guess these 5th graders that I went to school with were discovering the 999,871st, 2nd, 3rd, 4th and 5th digits? I'm guessing because I didn't care enough to ask why they voluntarily spent three months of their childhood on this quest. No judgment, but I was an average kid in comparison. The kids I went to school with have gone on to become Rhodes Scholars, master scientists, and chefs to the President of the United States #Obama. They are Oscar-winning screenwriters, and basically bosses of every shape and form.

My claim to fame in childhood was that my dad owned chains of fast food restaurants. In the 70s, my father, an accountant from West Virginia and a former CTA "El" train driver, went with a lawyer friend down to Louisiana to "taste some chicken." Hold on to your stereotypes. Everybody from all ethnicities "love[s] that Chicken from Popeye's." With the tantalizing taste and crunchy crust, a vision was born to introduce Chicago to this Louisiana gem. My father went on to own both Popeye's and Wendy's franchises, in addition to other sit- down and buffet-style restaurants. The recurrent theme of my childhood was being asked by countless strangers and new acquaintances if I got my name from the Wendy's restaurant. I became a Wendy's history and Dave Thomas scholar. I would respond with two facts: I was born before my father purchased the Wendy's franchise, and Dave Thomas himself had a daughter named Wendy. #wheresthebeef

At the end of the day, I was just an ordinary kid going to school with other somewhat ordinary kids, some of whose parents happened to own fortune 500 companies and mega hotel chains. Others had more regular families and backgrounds, like my crew of friends to this day. I considered it a bonus to be able to have lunch on a warm day as a high school senior at my dad's Wendy's, which was walking distance from my school. The best part was that I did not pay any money for the meal. All of the managers knew me.

I remember distinctly in my middle school years being considered weird. While I can't remember exactly how I got that distinction, I do remember one thing that I used to do that supported the diagnosis. I used to buy the little round cream cheese single-use container from the school cafeteria and, instead of buying a bagel to spread it on, I would just eat it. One cost 30 cents, and I would get a little disposable knife and eat it. That was weird to my friends. Now people eat crab Rangoon and cream cheese puffs like its natural. I just want to highlight that there is really no difference in what I did versus eating a hunk of cream cheese beneath a thin layer of fried pastry. My version actually had fewer calories.

To those who think that it must be disgusting to be an OB/GYN, I say that it is not. I am not at all grossed out by vaginas, most of the time. There are things that do gross me out though. But vaginas, blood, bowel movements, or funky feet didn't make it onto my list. As a mother, it isn't snot or vomit either. I'll catch throw-up bare handed without flinching #mompower. Here are my top 10 gross-outs. I hope you aren't eating while reading this.

1. Broken or dislocated bones and joints—we're talking a bad real- time sports injury. I shudder and get queasy with joints.

2. Animal smells. Not petting zoo stuff, but a funky dog or urine smell, especially in MY house. Bluh!

44

3. Things that make me itch. I'm talking about that creepy crawly feeling. A wool sweater digs into the depths of my soul. This aversion is actually why I don't shave my legs. The first time that I tried, it was an ambitious and misguided mission. I found my dad's face razor on my parent's sink and grabbed it, put some water on my legs, and shaved. Immediately that quest for girly glory turned into a burning sands Rights of Passage. My legs felt like I was being bitten by fire ants, or how I would imagine that it must feel. That itchy, burny madness scarred me for life. Thank God that my leg hair is fine and barely noticeable because if it weren't, I'd rock it anyway. Those itchy panel maternity pants that come up over the abdomen also irk me, the worst. They made me itch and instantly put me in a bad mood, not unlike many aspects of pregnancy. I rocked the under-belly elastic band maternity pants all of the way.

4. Public and visibly dirty showers, locker rooms, or gritty pool floors. I wear shower shoes to any tiled place outside my own home. There is something about the thought of grout grime, other people's hair, and clumps of what-is-that on tiled surfaces that make me want to gag. Seeing other people sport bare feet is equally disturbing to me.

5. Public toilets—seats, splashes, and flush mechanisms. I squat, flush and run. You are not going to spray me with whatever has taken residence in that public receptacle. The worst is when the door swings open toward the toilet and to get out, you need to back up toward the toilet, meanwhile the auto-flush has already begun, so you know you must be backing into the aerosol spray of all things nasty in the frantic effort to exit the stall with your life, health and dignity. I fight for that exit. I sometimes lose.

6. Bed bugs. (I think I have a phobia.) I check my sheets, mattress covers, pillows, pillowcases at every opportunity. Our mattresses have those anti-allergen and anti-bed bug covers. I've never seen one live and in person, and I know that they are not dangerous, just hard to get rid of. The thought still repulses me. I don't like any insect really, but in motherhood, I have gained a weird, what feels like primitive, protective nature. I used to run from a spider, but now I can take a deep breath and kill it with the psychological rationale that I am protecting my babies from its

45

babies. If I ever see a bed bug, I'll just have to grab the kids and run. Dear, insect rights people, I don't kill bugs unless they try to live where I live. If they are in nature I don't kill, and I teach my kids to leave them alone. In my house or car, though, if you don't pay rent or insurance, you gotta go. That would apply to anyone.

7. Dirty fingernails. Cut and scrub, please. Yuck.

8. Bare-hand baby delivery. I have always said that, with rare exception, a term (old enough to deliver) baby cannot come out too fast. I am speaking strictly in regards to baby safety. As an OB/GYN, I can think of countless things that can go wrong during a delivery. Many of the issues that can compromise the safety and long-term well-being of an infant have to do with what happens in the home stretch of labor because of baby's oxygenation, issues with getting stuck during a vaginal delivery, or difficulties during a cesarean section (C-section.) If a term baby just flies out unexpectedly in the hospital waiting room, on the highway on the way to the hospital, or on the bathroom floor of your house or Walmart, they may make a mess and cause everyone to freak out, but generally, that baby will be fine. If I am there as this baby is making an unexpectedly rapid entrance into this world, be ready for me to grab something to catch the baby in. Give up your clothes, headwrap, something. I don't mind blood and guts, but I will not have all of that mixed with vagina juice touch my bare hands if I can help it.

9. People who touch their private areas and then other parts of their body or other items without washing their hands. Who would do that? So many people, you don't even know. If you want to show me a new lump or bump, pretend I am on the phone and you are trying to direct me to your house. "What street do you see? Okay, turn left, drive down two blocks. Do you see the green house with the fence? I'm the next house." Vagina version: "Okay, it's on my left outer labia. No, lower than that. Do you see the inner area right where the hair stops growing? It is little, white and about the size of the end of a pen." I can follow directions and find it. Don't reach down there and feel around and then proceed to pick up your phone, fix your hair and touch my doorknob on the way out with your unwashed vagina-hand. I know it's what I do for a living, but I

wash my hands upon entry and exit of every room and I wear gloves before I touch anything. I realize it's yours, but don't touch and then spread that love everywhere.

10. A tampon that has been in the vagina way too long. As a teenager, I read that toxic shock syndrome would happen if you left your tampon in too long. I remember worrying if I would be okay if I left mine in overnight. Turns out that that was the least of my worries. There is nothing (or at least very few things) more foul smelling than a lost and forgotten tampon. I go into toxic shock when I have to go on a search and recovery mission for a tampon that has been in place for days or weeks. It's not the thought of it that repulses me. No judgment against any of the ladies who I have freed from tampon retention in my career. You are fine women and it can happen to anyone. The problem is that they smell so, so, SO bad. Think of something that you know smells terrible. Old raw chicken parts, spoiled eggs, dog poop. A retained tampon is worse. I don't walk into those moments with a smile, or at least not a real one. As the old adage says, it's a dirty job, but somebody has to do it.

Even though I have no problem being in contact with vaginas of all backgrounds, ages, and conditions on a daily basis, I have two basic requirements to do my job: soap and running water. There was once a time when the building that houses my office had a mechanical failure that caused the water pumps to go out. Here we were, getting a building-wide memo that said "the facilities will still be opened, and we have power. Please carry on with business as usual or work from home." I responded, "Do they know what we do? I cannot (and wouldn't want to) do what I do from home, and business as usual without water is a no-go for me."

I saw pregnant patients and anyone who needed only a verbal consultation. I'll use hand sanitizer after I shake someone's hand or touch their pregnant abdomen. There is no sanitizer in the world that will mentally cleanse me from being involved with someone's lady parts. I promptly rescheduled any visit that involved vaginas until the water returned. I guess if the world as we know it ends and we lose power and running water, I may need to find another career. I'm guessing that I won't be the only one.

3
LET THE ALPHABETICAL GOOD TIMES ROLL

D.

Dementia

"Y'all gon' make me lose my mind up in here, up in here."
A song that sounded so #urbandictionary "hard" back in '99, reads so corny in this chapter.

Dementia is a general term that refers to a decline in mental processes that can affect memory, personality, reasoning and general capacity for normal activities of daily living. Alzheimer's is one type, but dementia can also arise from physical trauma, chronic disease and just basic aging. As much as I would love to be one of those ladies who in their 80s or 90s is "sharp as a tack", if my brain function right now is any predictor, I may be off of solid foods and wearing a diaper by 70. God be with me.

An important part of dementia is personality changes. My father used to refer to my grandmother, his mother-in-law, as cantankerous. Not an abnormal sentiment for some sons-in-law regarding their MIL, but in this situation, I think the primary reason she was so progressively grumpy and hard to deal with was her brain degeneration. Over time, she stopped eating well, drinking enough fluids, and she would forget to go to the restroom when needed. If we didn't know that her brain function was slowly deteriorating, it would have been hard to accept her banter.

The take-home message here is to know that some of our elders with dementia aren't "mean" just to annoy us. It is their brain that is not working well. I pray that mine keeps working, or if it slows to a halt before I make my "transition", I pray for patient caretakers and loved ones who I won't have to burden, God willing, for too long.

Dental Health

There are a surprising number of correlates between good dental hygiene and general health. The teeth and gums are an access point for bacteria. Without regular brushing, flossing, and periodic dental check-ups, the body's defenses are easily breached right inside of your mouth. Pregnancy is a particularly vulnerable time when the teeth are an unsuspecting source of risk to mother and child.

During pregnancy, your risk of gum disease and cavity development, also known as tooth decay, goes up. There is also legitimate data that suggests risks of preterm labor and other pregnancy complications may be related to some degree to poor dental health. Periodontal disease is an inflammatory disease that affects the soft and hard structures that support the teeth. In its early stage, called gingivitis, the gums become swollen and red due to inflammation, which is the body's natural response to the presence of harmful bacteria. The theory is that gum disease and tooth decay increase the amount of bacteria that make it into a mother's bloodstream and also increases her overall amount of inflammation in the body. This can affect the unborn fetus and can cause low birth weight and preterm labor.

The American Dental Association makes the following recommendations: Brush your teeth twice a day with a soft-bristled brush. The size and shape of your brush should fit your mouth allowing you to reach all areas easily. Replace your toothbrush every three or four months, or sooner if the bristles are frayed. A worn toothbrush won't do a good job of cleaning your teeth. Make sure to use an ADA-accepted fluoride toothpaste. The proper brushing technique is to place your toothbrush at a 45-degree angle to the gums. Gently move the brush back and forth in short (tooth-wide) strokes. Brush the outer surfaces, the inner surfaces, and the chewing surfaces of the teeth. To clean the inside surfaces of the front teeth, tilt the brush vertically and make several up-and-down strokes.

One thing that the dental hygienist at my dentist's office shared with me is that it doesn't matter what time of day you floss. I always thought that you had to floss at the same time that you brush. While there isn't anything wrong with that practice, it is also okay to floss while just sitting on the couch watching TV. As long as you don't fling little between-the-teeth food particles around my living room, I support increasing the opportunities to improve dental hygiene.

Deodorant

There is no conclusive evidence that aluminum containing deodorant causes breast cancer or any cancer. There are conflicting data and a lot of speculation, so caution is not wrong. I cannot recommend that everyone stop using mainstream aluminum-containing deodorants, though, without sound evidence. Do I in my own bathroom have aluminum free "natural" deodorant? Yes, right next to my real deal, it's-gonna-be-an-intense-and-possibly-funky-day aluminum containing deodorant.

Depression

See Body Blues. Sorry for the redirect this time. The D's were saturated.

Diaphragm

See Contraceptives. Yes, some ladies still use these, in case you were wondering.

Diastasis Recti

This is a pregnancy phenomenon that is worthy of a section because of the anxiety that it causes. Diastasis Recti (also known as abdominal separation) is commonly defined as a significant gap between the two sides of the rectus abdominis, or middle ab muscle. This condition does not cause actual physical harm in most cases. It happens sometimes in pregnancy. Hernias may be more likely to form when diastasis is present. Physical therapy can sometimes reduce the degree of separation and improve it. If it doesn't bother you (by its appearance or otherwise), it doesn't bother me. My own diastasis recti doesn't bother me, so I'm not insensitive to the subject.

Discharge

There are so many different things that can come out of a woman's vagina—from babies to blood, to urine, though urine is not technically from the vagina (see Anatomy). The vagina can be mysterious and difficult to control. A common question in my office is, "What is going on with my discharge?" The first thing that I want to make clear is that the epithelium of the vagina is moist for a reason. It is meant to lubricate and keep the communication between the outside world and the uterus well-guarded. There are different types of bacteria that are supposed to be there, as well as white blood cells. On any given day, the secretions within this personal space can be abundant or minimal, but they can still be normal.

Different things can affect the quality and quantity of discharge. With normal discharge, hormonal fluctuations related to ovulation and an impending menstrual cycle can cause this fluid to be milky, or clear and slimy, or thicker and yellowish. There isn't a discharge key that applies to every woman, but ovulation does, for most women, yield a clear slippery discharge that is meant to aid in sperm transport through the cervix. Remember, every ovulation is a potential pregnancy for your body, whether you like it or not. If you have made the decision to prevent pregnancy with combined estrogen-progesterone containing oral contraceptives, you won't ovulate (assuming proper use), but this can also change your discharge. I have even had women who thought that their discharge was abnormal because it changed in consistency after stopping birth control. Your on-birth-control vagina is often different from your off-birth-control vagina.

Pregnancy can also change discharge. Although that too is different for every woman, the general consensus from most women is that discharge increases in quantity during pregnancy. The call that I sometimes get is, "Did my bag of water break?" I never scoff at a woman for asking that question. Rupture of membranes, as it is called in the OB/GYN world, is serious, especially in a preterm pregnancy. My general rule of thumb for a woman without a classic movie-like gush of water that soaks her clothes and splashes on the floor like the end of the dance scene in Flashdance is that if it goes past your underwear, it warrants evaluation. That means, if a woman's underwear is damp only, it is likely just the extra juices and berries (surprise Coming to America reference) that come from gestating a human. If her pants or dress or pajamas or bed also have a wet spot, no matter how small, at the very least her doctor should be called and included in the conversation about whether or not to evaluate. Call your doctor though if you are ever concerned.

Characteristics that can signal a discharge problem, even in pregnancy, are itching, irritation and odor. My first question when I prepare for a vaginal exam is, "Is there any concern for an STD?" "Any concern" can be something as simple as having had a new sexual partner. I don't ask because I think every discharge is caused by a disease, but I never put it past a vagina to have something unwelcome and I want to give every woman an opportunity to be evaluated. I have been in practice for over 10 years and I have never called someone to inform them that they had an STD who said, "Oh, I knew I had that!" It is ALWAYS a surprise, with the rare exception of the woman who found out her partner was cheating when they told her that they had contracted a disease. Even then, it is not always a given that the disease was passed to my patient, but in that situation, we treat presumptively while we wait for the test results.

Once we get past the STD question and/or test, I am looking for ulcerations, signs of inflammation, or a foul odor. I test for common culprits like yeast and bacterial vaginosis. I also check for and ask about new exposures to products like fragranced soaps, detergents, fabric softeners, vaginal lubricants, or anything that the sensitive skin of the vagina may not like. Urinary evaluation is also reasonable. Sometimes the burn of a urinary tract infection can be confused for the burn of a bad yeast infection. Read more about yeast in the Candidiasis section.

I have to say again that discharge can be normal. The glands within the vagina and the cervix secrete, well, secretions. Sometimes one can correlate those secretions with the time in one's cycle or a level of arousal. If it doesn't itch or have an odor, and your concern for sexually transmitted infections is low, it isn't unreasonable to just keep an eye on it and track symptoms in a chart or calendar. A completely dry or discharge-free vagina isn't the goal either. Actually, my peri-menopausal and post-menopausal women will vouch for the desire to have a little more moisture in that region. A dry vagina is not comfortable.

Let's talk more about Bacterial Vaginosis now.

Bacterial Vaginosis reminds me of the fresh aroma of Lake Michigan Perch. My dad used to go fishing on random Saturday and Sunday mornings in Lake Michigan. He would bring home a 3-gallon bucket full of Perch or other types of fish. This was back in the '80s and early '90s. There was nothing fishier than the kitchen that housed that bucket...except maybe a strong case of Bacterial Vaginosis. Did you know that in medical school we were taught to use the Whiff Test to aid in the diagnosis of BV? If you put a dab of discharge on a slide, and drop some Potassium Hydroxide, or KOH, on the slide, the cells on the slide break apart, and an amine smell wafts up to slap you in your nares. It smells like fish. What other medical diagnosis does smell aid in arriving at the proper diagnosis? Maybe gangrene.

The diagnosis is made with either a microscopic slide evaluation or a culture or DNA probe. The treatment can be antibiotics or, one of my new favorites, Boric Acid vaginal suppositories. Talk to your gynecologist about your options, especially if you are getting these infections frequently. Vaginas misbehave in various ways that are a little too broad for you to be able to use this book to diagnose. You can always try dietary changes (like less sugar), boric acid suppositories, and specific vaginal probiotics. The problem with a vaginal infection is that it is really hard to diagnose which one you are dealing with without testing. I don't know what women did before gynecologists. Itched and smelled, I guess.

Double-Dutch Vagina Syndrome

I know what you are thinking.

"I didn't know that you can get a syndrome from jumping Double-Dutch."

Well, DDVS is not some weird chaffing like the kind that I am told is caused by long runs or bike rides. Actually, it is not a REAL syndrome at all. This is an original term that I like to use to refer to times when a woman can't seem to hold onto a healthy, normal smelling, appropriate or no discharge, itch-free vagina. One moment it is bothering you, and you want to take it off your body completely. The next moment you take meds or change habits, and you think it's better, just good enough to use (smh), but then it's back acting up again. It's never out of the shop long enough to get you on that road trip you've been planning.

If you've ever jumped Double Dutch, you know that timing is key. You need to jump in at the perfect time; otherwise, you may just get slapped in the face by the ropes or end up on the ground, embarrassed. DDVS is similar in that if you don't catch the healthy, comfortable, sweet smelling vagina just right, you will be uncomfortable, in pain, or just have to make up an off-limits excuse for any hanky-panky. To all of the Marvin Gayes out there, sexual healing doesn't apply here. When she gets THAT feeling, she needs... you to keep your distance. What is the remedy for DDVS? Evaluation and treatment, just like any other set of symptoms prior to confirming the diagnosis. I don't have a one-med-treats-all answer. I just like the DDVS concept and wanted to share it with my readers. Well, I don't really LIKE the concept, I just like putting a name to a face. Feel free to hashtag, though you may not want to publicize your DDVS status on social media...or...anywhere. #makeanappointment #DDVS

Douching

I don't curse, but the word "douche" may as well be a 4-letter word in a gynecologist's office. The word douche means (1) a spray of water, or (2) An obnoxious or contemptible person (typically used of a man). You gotta love number two! In the realm of gynecology, douching is the practice of washing or flushing the vagina with water or other fluids. Vaginal douches most commonly involving water mixed with vinegar, baking soda, or iodine. I have even seen stainless steel douche systems where a stainless steel wand is connected to the sink faucet and used to deodorize and flush the vagina with water in the same way that the steel kitchen faucet can deodorize your oniony hands when cooking. I also had a patient recently tell me she douches with diluted peroxide to decrease her frequency of developing bacterial vaginosis. #dontdothat

So what's the problem with it? I'm glad you asked. The vagina is supposed to have bacteria in it. A certain composition of bacteria at the appropriate ratios is to be expected and is healthy. The words clean and vagina are relatively oxymoronic—the vagina is just not a clean place. Let me take a moment to be clear. I am talking about the inside of the vagina. The outside can also harbor odor that no douche in the world can fix. That takes the right kind of soap and water, and likely some gentle grooming. Excessive hair can hold odor and oils that can keep the crotch smelling pungent. I like electric trimmers as a do-it-yourself painless way to keep your personal lawn mowed. Evidence shows that douching increases the frequency of bacterial infections of the vagina. Ironic, huh. That means that the process of using douche to achieve a "cleaner" vagina for the improvement of its smell, or for the benefit of a partner, can lead to the opposite effect of more frequent and more severe infections. Tell your partner that it's not supposed to smell like roses. Now if it smells like popcorn, we may have something to talk about.

A myth that has been disproven is that there is no increase in the risks of ectopic pregnancy and pelvic inflammatory disease in women who douche over women who don't. Is the vagina a self-cleaning oven? Yes. Does that oven sometimes get a little scorched and need a little Easy-off? Maybe. Some methods to reset the pH when things seem to get out of balance are a pH balanced gel, boric acid suppositories, and pelvic rest (i.e. no sex). A mild scent is often very normal. There may even be a pheromone component to the smell in the nether-region. The main thing to remember is that if you think your smell is not normal or if you are uncomfortable, see your gynecologist rather than that drug-store squeeze bottle.

Dr. Every Woman

Dr. Every Woman is the part of me that feels connected to every woman. All of us have something special. We sing in the car, or we have crazy kids, or we care about our health, or we have a hard time keeping our house clean, or we want our kids to be more confident, or we love our husbands, but they get under our skin as no one else can. In a world where perfection is the facade of every reality show or Hollywood personality, Dr. Every Woman represents the fact that we all have challenges in life, but sometimes those challenges are more common than we think. We all are different and we should celebrate both our differences and our similarities. My goal is to normalize the things that make us different, similar and special.

This marks the beginning of the Every Woman Movement. This movement means that we each celebrate each other's accomplishments, but seek to reduce each other's pitfalls. We also care about and want to change injustices when they affect anyone, especially women and children around the world. You are Every

Woman if you hope to see every man, woman and child treated fairly and removed from the crippling weight of oppression.

Due Date

I'm sprinkling pregnancy pearls throughout this book because childbearing is an integral part of women's health as a whole, even if every woman doesn't have a baby. Bear with me if these topics don't apply to you personally, but I challenge you to read them anyway because you never know when a topic you've learned about can actually help a pregnant woman. I stress the ACTUALLY HELP part because, this may come as a surprise, but a lot of information voluntarily shared with pregnant women by friends and family doesn't actually help them. If you don't believe me, here are some examples:

Exhibit A: "When are you due? Oh, you are so big/small. You might have that baby [prematurely] this week."

Exhibit B: "Let me tell you about my super dramatic and traumatic labor story, even though it will not save you from any misfortune or add to your safety at all. It will, however, increase your anxiety through the roof."

So the age-old truth that we OB/GYNs know, but confuse pregnant moms with, is the correlation between a baby's size, baby's age, and mom's due date. Early on, the baby's size and the mom's last period are used to determine when the baby is due. Based on the classic last menstrual period calculation, a woman is already 2 weeks pregnant before she even has sex. That little revelation has brought down many a raised eyebrow from a partner who finds out: "She is 6 weeks pregnant? But we had sex 4 weeks ago!" Yes, fellas, we count from the period, which is 2 weeks before she even released that egg. Call it crazy but those are the rules.

Now back to this size discussion. If the initial ultrasound in the first trimester measures the baby to be the same size as the gestational age calculated by the last menstrual period (LMP), give or take less than a week, the due date based on the last menstrual period is established. Example time: Your LMP says you are 7 weeks pregnant with a due date of August 10th. The ultrasound says you are 7 weeks and 2 days pregnant with a due date of August 8th. That is within 1 week and can be explained by a margin of ultrasound not-exactness (I made that term up), so you are 7 weeks pregnant with a due date of August 10th. If the ultrasound said you are 8 weeks with a due date of August 3rd, there is discrepancy that likely means you ovulated early. We would then adjust the due date to August 3rd.

Once the due date has been established and confirmed, with ultrasound if possible, it now becomes a marker for the baby's age. We will use it to say, "Now you are 20 weeks pregnant or 30 weeks pregnant." The countdown to the due date determines how long the baby has been growing. Now say a mom's belly is measuring, yes MEASURING (not just looking big to your untrained and unsolicited eye) larger than normal. In that situation, we order an ultrasound. Let's say the baby does appear to be a little larger than normal for this gestational age on ultrasound. Well, just like if your toddler is in the 90th percentile for size, that doesn't change their age, a fetus in the uterus doesn't all of a sudden get older and "want to come out sooner" because they are bigger. Your big or small baby is just that—big or small. Sometimes in extreme situations, a baby may need to be delivered based on why and to what degree they are big or small, but that is only when their health is in question. Imagine though, that you plant a bunch of seeds in a garden. In the beginning, all of the seedlings will be the same size. In time, though, some plants will grow more than others. They are all the same age though.

A due date does not determine exactly when a baby will be born in most circumstances. A few exceptions to that rule are women who have scheduled C-sections or inductions (induced labor) for pregnancy complications like diabetes. What the due date DOES establish is how old a baby is. Most babies take about 40 weeks to "cook" or "percolate." No, the baby isn't a turkey or a pot of coffee, but the entire process of bringing the single egg and sperm cells to a functional baby that can be born and survive with enough fat to keep him or her warm and with a mature nervous system to regulate blood sugars and mature organs to breathe unassisted etc. takes about 40 weeks from the last menstrual period. I bring up those specific functions, because when babies are born early, especially less than 37 weeks (which is the definition of premature), these and other functions may not work very well. Think of that before you tell the next pregnant woman who looks "big" that "That baby is going to come early." Bite your tongue and let that baby percolate. #imfromchicago #thepercolatorwasadance.

The take-home message: Baby size helps to establish a due date at the beginning of pregnancy. Once that date is established, your baby is just big or small. Work with your doctor to determine if there are any implications based on your baby's size. Finally, STOP telling pregnant women that you know or meet randomly that they look big or small. You are messing with their emotions, and then I have to calm them down. STOP IT! 😊

E.

Ectopic Pregnancy

This topic was touched on previously in the Anatomy section under Fallopian Tube. That is because the most common type of ectopic pregnancy is one of tubal origin. There are different locations where an ectopic pregnancy can be present. The definition of an ectopic pregnancy is a pregnancy that conceives and implants outside of the uterus. Here are some little known ectopic pregnancy facts:

1.   A pregnancy can implant in the tube, cornua (corner of the uterus), cervix, ovary, or abdomen.

2.   Ectopic pregnancies are often diagnosed in early stages with a common symptom being bleeding and/or pain.

3.   These pregnancies can sometimes be treated with a medication called methotrexate in single or multiple doses but sometimes need surgery.

4.   Women with a history of sexually transmitted disease, especially pelvic inflammatory disease, are at increased risk for having this type of pregnancy.

5.   Women who use IUDs for birth control are not at increased risks of having an ectopic pregnancy over the general population. They do have a relative increase in ectopic pregnancy in that since any intra-uterine pregnancy is so uncommon, if a pregnancy were to occur in that less than one percent scenario, that pregnancy may be outside of the uterus, or ectopic.

Ectopic pregnancies do not often resolve on their own and can be life-threatening. They are so dangerous because of the brisk and perfuse blood loss that can occur if one ruptures. Don't sleep. In fact, there is a saying in the OB/GYN world: "Never let the sun set on a bleeding ectopic." These are not "Let's operate tomorrow" types of surgeries, but rather more like "When can we go back to the

OR (operating room)?" no matter what time it is types of surgeries. If it has happened to you once, there is a higher likelihood that it will happen again. Anyone who has a history of ectopic pregnancy should be followed super closely from the moment that they find out that they are pregnant to make sure it isn't another ectopic. I feel like I am due for a good joke, but this subject doesn't evoke much humor from me. Though I have never had one, I see women who I am grateful to see alive despite this dangerous diagnosis. These same women are understandably devastated that they lost the life they had been yearning for in order to save their own. Many of these women go on to have healthy babies after ectopics, but some don't and that is so sad. Uh, what is the next topic?

Embolization

Uterine artery embolization (UAE) is a way to control heavy bleeding that is caused by benign structures like large fibroids. During a UAE, a radiologist feeds a catheter through one of the blood vessels in your groin. Then after advancing that catheter to the level of the blood vessels that feed the uterus, small beads are released that block and cut off much of the blood supply to the uterus and the fibroids. This procedure should shrink the uterus by 30% and slow or stop blood loss from the uterus. Much like hysteroscopic ablation, this is not always a permanent fix. Pregnancy after embolization is discouraged, though it is not considered birth control. A pregnancy after a UAE can lead to miscarriage or abnormal placental attachment, among other pregnancy complications. Lock down that birth control, ladies.

Endometriosis

Endometriosis is one of those diseases that many people have, but few people know about. In the article "Endometriosis: Ancient Disease, Ancient Treatments," published by Camran Nezhat et al. the history of endometriosis was chronicled. The best part about the article was when they uncovered evidence that many cases of "hysteria," the female-only psychological disorder of the olden days, may well have been endometriosis all along:
Several other disease profiles from pre-modern times were also identified for the first time as sharing striking similarities with

endometriosis symptoms, including the so-called disease of virgins, lovesickness, furor uterinus (uterine fury), strangulation of the womb, suffocation of the womb, catamenial hematoceles, and many more.

What did that just say? Well, pretty much that historically, women with Endo were thought to be crazy. Like women needed endometriosis to be crazy! Just kidding.

Endometriosis is a hard diagnosis to make. It can cause pain without any ultrasonographic signs of disease. I have recently begun (like in the last 10 minutes) referring to endometriosis as the Keyser Soze of the pelvis. Remember that dude in the movie The Usual Suspects who seemed all innocent and flew under the radar, but ended up being the ONE responsible for the whole fiasco? A person can have severe pain and a completely normal ultrasound, but Endo can be the cause. Conversely, a woman can have a lot of endometriosis in the pelvis seen at the time of surgery and yet have very little symptoms. The amount or extent of disease and the severity of a woman's symptoms don't always correlate with one another.

So how is the diagnosis made and what do you do about it? The only way to definitively make the diagnosis is to biopsy lesions during surgery and send them for pathology. If the pathologist sees hemosiderin-laden macrophages, voila, you have your diagnosis. I know you must be thinking that you were told, or your friend or auntie was told that they have it and they never had surgery or a biopsy. That is because we usually make the diagnosis based on symptoms. We call that empiric diagnosis. If I suspect the diagnosis based on your story (which we docs call your history) and physical exam, I can try to treat it. If the treatment or management works, then I can feel confident that I made the right diagnosis. If it doesn't, I may need to keep digging.

A classic management of endometriosis symptoms is the use of birth control pills or anything that prevents ovulation. Endo causes pain because of the cyclic bleeding of the implants within your pelvis. Whatever can stop ovulation can also stop that cyclic bleeding and pain.

Endometriosis implants are basically little unwelcome patches of uterine lining that end up in places other than the inside of the uterus. How those implants got outside of the uterus is anyone's guess, but when they bleed, they can cause pain in the pelvis and/or cysts on the ovaries. There are many medical theories about the "How did this happen?" question. The conclusion of those theories about how the implants got to their extrauterine locations is basically—no one really knows. Birth control pills prevent them from bleeding as much, if at all, by decreasing their hormonal food that comes from our brains naturally. Over time, they get smaller and less problematic, but after the ovulation controlling agent is removed, they can return.

I often get asked, "Well isn't the pill just masking the symptoms?" Yes, in some ways it is. In other ways, it is like depriving weeds of water so they shrivel up and die. I am all about tackling the source of a problem when that is realistic. In this case, tackling the source isn't very realistic unless a person is trying to conceive and is having trouble, or she is having severe pain that is not improved with our non-surgical options. Unless a woman is in either of those scenarios, we would be doing many unnecessary surgeries if we operated on everyone with suspected endometriosis. Surgery is the only definitive treatment but shouldn't be done too often.

As I just mentioned, Endo can affect fertility but doesn't always. Laparoscopic surgery may be required to evaluate and treat endometriosis if fertility appears to be compromised and other causes of infertility are ruled out. Other treatments of endometriosis include GNRH agonists and antagonists, which shut down the hormonal food from the brain by putting a woman into a temporary menopausal state. Another is the hormonal birth control implant that goes into the arm. It also stops ovulation, which should improve symptoms and ideally shrink endometriosis over time.

Epidural

Epidural anesthesia, or an epidural, is only the best thing since babies were invented. The term actually refers to the space in a person's back where pain medication can be injected to numb a person's legs and abdomen. I have had three of these in my lifetime because I have three babies and personally, I wasn't about that pain-med free birth life. No judgment against women who want to or have done this. You ladies are stronger than I am. No really, you are stronger than I am. I took the drugs.

A few misconceptions to highlight:
    1. Though a needle is used to enter the spinal column area,

no needle is left in the back. Only a small flexible plastic catheter is left behind in the back to deliver a continuous infusion of pain medication.

2. The place where the catheter is placed is beneath the spinal cord where all of the nerves live, so paralysis is a near impossibility.

3. The labor course may be slowed by getting an epidural too early, but the C-section rate is not significantly affected by this change in pace. I had three vaginal deliveries. If my labor was slowed by a few hours, that's cool with me. Those were some pain-free extra hours.

4. Scheduled C-sections don't often require an epidural. A spinal dose of directly injected medication usually will last for more than enough time to finish a cesarean delivery. No catheter is needed.

5. Epidurals are safe for babies. I practice at a hospital where over ten thousand babies are born every year, and more than ninety percent of women get epidurals. If epidurals were out here causing harm to moms or babies, I and the general public would know about it.

Some can get a spinal headache after an epidural. The anesthesiologists know how to treat this better than I. What I do know is that this happens infrequently and is temporary. I will end this section with yet another original hashtag: #Thereisnoshameinnopain

Exercise

Despite my size, I am in no way a fitness fanatic. I get my muscle tone from my dad, who has the calves of a warrior, but I am what is known as skinny fat. I'm not self-deprecating. Skinny fat is a thing. I am not the traditional type of skinny fat where I lack lean muscle and have disproportionately too much fat in the way that some do. I don't have a lot of body fat. My vice is that I don't have the cardiovascular health that I need. Put me on too many flights of stairs, and I'll become Redd Fox from Sandford and Son: "I'm comin' home."

Cardiovascular health is important. The goal for maintaining your current weight is 150 minutes of moderate exercise per week, or 75 minutes of intense exercise per week. Keep in mind, this is only the exercise portion of weight maintenance. Don't think that if you adhere to these guidelines, you also can eat whatever you want or drink sugar to your heart's content. You are lying to yourself. Assuming a reasonable diet, primarily plant-based, water-rich, lean-meat full diet, 150 minutes of light cardio or 75 minutes of boot camp-ishness should keep you steady.

Now if you are trying to lose weight, first change your diet. A whole workout can be negated with ONE MEAL, especially from any fast food chain of your choice. Once you have changed your diet, you are looking at 300 minutes of exercise per week to start losing. Before you get all in a tizzy convincing yourself of how impossible that is, try this. I borrowed this plan from my husband. Work out for 1 hour on Saturday and Sunday. That is 120 minutes. Then get 30 minutes per day during the week. That makes 270. That's close enough in my book (no pun intended). If you are a stickler though, just add 10 minutes to 3 of the 5 daily workouts, and voila. Sidebar: voila is French for "there it is." Some try to spell it vuala, but that's wrong. #sorrynotsorry #idontspeakfrench. #idospeakspanishfluently #thisiscalledoverhashtagging #ijustmadethatup.

I want to close this topic with a petition to let my trip to Costco count as a workout. Tom Joyner had a nationally syndicated radio show where he was always making certain appearances and experiences "count" as church. Like a gospel brunch or a religious radio guest, if they said anything that led in any way to spiritual growth, he would say "I think that counts as church." The point was that he was now exempt from having to go to "actual church" that week. Well, I think my trip to Costco should "count" as a workout for the following reasons:

1. I'm reluctant to unload my cart, empty my car, or go to the superstore altogether.

2. I can easily work up a sweat.

3. I regret bringing my kids because they are a distraction and slow me down.

4.I paid for the Costco membership so I feel like I should use it, much like a gym membership.

5. I get hungry and thirsty during and after my trip.

6. There are definitely some squats and snatches involved.

7. Reps are a thing when loading and unloading items.

8. I am very self-conscious until I realize that we are all

carrying around weight that we don't need.

Today's workout? CHECK!

F.

FACOG

FACOG stands for Fellow of the American College of Obstetrics and Gynecology. A doctor can only get this distinction after they pass an obnoxiously long slew of tests to become certified by the American Board of Obstetricians and Gynecologists. Because I passed ALL of those tests, I am board-certified. Every year, I have to maintain that certification with continued education. If you have ever wondered what it takes to become a doctor, and specifically a board-certified OB/GYN, wonder no longer. Let's take it from the top:

1. Elementary school. 8 years. I'm a product of the University of Chicago Laboratory Schools.

2. High, or Secondary, school. High School Diploma. 4 years. Still a Labbie for me (that's what we called ourselves).

3. College or University. Bachelor's Degree in something. Interestingly, you don't need a Bachelor's degree in the sciences to become a doctor. Docs with English degrees actually have been shown to do better in medicine because of all of the writing we have to do. My B.S. is a Bachelor's of Science from the amazing Xavier University of Louisiana. #xurocksthehouse. 4 years (or however long it takes you to get that degree). Sidebar: Is it too feminist to wonder if there should be a Bachelorette's degree?

4. Medical school: Either Allopathic or Osteopathic. One is no better or worse than the other, just different in their focuses. Both are comprehensive. I am an Allopath from Northwestern University Feinberg School of Medicine. Osteopaths are D.O.s instead of M.D.s. 4 years (or however long it takes you to get that degree). Some do combined MD/JD, MD/MBA, or MD/PhD programs which take longer but have value in their own right.

5. USMLE Step 1, Step 2 and Step 3 are intense and expensive national exams required to graduate from medical school.

6. Residency: 3-5 years depending on the specialty. OB/GYN is 4 years. Subspecialties in OB/GYN can add 1-3 years on top of that. Generally speaking, the ABOG written exam is taken during residency. Yet another grey hair producing, sleep depriving, financially draining exam that we have to take to prove that we won't be out here practicing in a non-standard way.

7. After 2-6 years of being in practice post-residency, and after the ABOG written exam is passed, enter the dreaded Oral Board exams. This is a 3-hour exam where we sit in front of two examiners and are drilled with questions about our management of patients we cared for over the year prior to the exam as well as general knowledge. FOR three straight hours. Many a blouse armpit has been ruined during this exam. Thousands of hours and dollars are spent preparing for this exam. If you don't pass it, you cannot claim "Board Certified" on anything. No, Ikea furniture assembly proficiency doesn't count for this board certification. No? Not funny? I thought that one was pretty good.

8. Lastly, you have now passed your boards and continue your yearly maintenance of certification. Now you need to pay those ACOG annual dues to be considered a Fellow of the American…well you know what it's called. No offense, ACOG, ABOG or any other board of anything that I am a part of or am certified by. Don't revoke my status. I worked too hard, paid too much, and am too traumatized to have to do it all over again. I'd need a new career. I'd be like a doc from another country who refuses to repeat all of their training to be able to practice in the U.S. When is the next The Voice audition? #imnotthatgood

Feminism

My girl Merriam Webster (I know Merriam-Webster isn't a woman, but for the purposes of this topic, let's pretend) defines feminism as the belief that men and women should have equal rights and opportunities. Merriam also says that feminism often relates to organized activity in support of women's rights and interests. Over the years, feminism has garnered a bad rap, even among women, for being too victimizing or exclusionary to men. I am a proud feminist. I believe that women and men should have equal rights. I'll tell you who else are feminists: my husband, my male OB/GYN partner, and probably most men who I associate with, whether they self-identify as such or not.

Much like the Black Lives Matter movement, which is pro-equal treatment and anti-discriminatory abuse of Black and Brown people, being pro-BLM, doesn't equate to being anti-everyone-else. My belief in my own rights as an African-American person, and as a woman, doesn't lead me to want to diminish the rights of anyone else. The idea that to be pro-one-thing means that you have to be anti-the-opposite-or-complimentary-thing is flawed. In a marriage, I want my husband to treat me as his equal, not better than himself. I want my kids to each have their own self-confidence and courage but not be bullies. In fact, in my household, my sons at one point would be sad if I didn't give them both the same compliment. We had to change that to a culture where if I give one a compliment, the other reinforces it with an honest and sincere compliment as well.

For example:
    Me: "Son, you did great on your spelling test."
    Other son: "Good job, brother. Keep it up."
    First son: "Thanks, brother. That was nice."
    Second son: "Thanks for saying thanks."
    First son: "Thanks for saying, 'Thanks for saying thanks.'"

And it would go on and on until I would break it up. They thought it was hilarious. I thought it was way better than the previous "Aww, did I do well on my spelling test too?"

    If I say, "Women should be able to make their own decisions about their bodies without interference from spouses, parents, and the government," I don't expect men to say. "Aww, don't I have rights to make my own decisions too?" Of course, men should have the same rights. That response would sound ridiculous if it were to be said out loud. Be feminist proud, man, woman and child. Hell, my dog better be a feminist if he wants me to take him out (when my husband can't, of course). If he is nice, he will probably even get a longer walk and a treat out of his adventures with me. He just needs to learn how to say "women's rights" in

Scooby Doo voice. I'm a softie. Sidebar: I would be a masculinist if a large scale movement began to foster equal and fair rights for men. I'm an equal opportunity advocate for what's right.

Fertility

Defined, fertility is the ability to conceive children. Fertility begins in puberty for both men and women. For women, the rates of successful pregnancy start to slowly decline within the late 20s and early 30s. Simultaneously, the changes in the rate of pregnancy complications and chromosomally or otherwise abnormal children go up with age. What that translates into is lower chances of getting pregnant and higher risk pregnancies the older we get. Patients often ask about their own risks in the setting of approaching 35 years old. 35 is not a magical age. It is not a proverbial cliff that a woman ages up to and then drops her eggs off the side of.

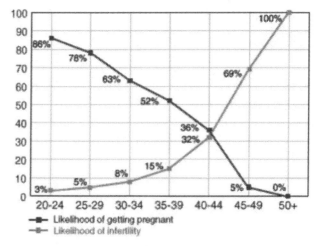

Source: https://www.babycenter.com

Sometimes I have to tell a woman whose ovaries have stopped functioning that they are essentially infertile. I never say never, but a woman with hormone levels suggesting premature ovarian failure or early menopause is likely going to be facing the need for egg donation if she wants to have any reasonable chance of getting pregnant. A less reliable test result is one that suggests normal fertility. The best possible test for fertility is an attempt to get pregnant. If that isn't feasible, tests that indicate normal hormone levels and uterine structure still in no way guarantee a person's success when she tries to conceive. There are so many factors affecting fertility, many of which we have no real handle on. A person with a history of infertility or pelvic disease can still sometimes become pregnant spontaneously. Conversely, a woman with a completely normal test for tubal patency (which confirms that the fallopian tubes are opened), normal uterus, normal hormones, and normal sperm (Yes, we test the men too!) can still have unexplained infertility.

While I don't discourage women from getting "fertility tests" when they aren't actively trying to conceive, I try to tell them not to rely completely on those results, even if they are normal. To my 28 and 30-year-olds who think they are old, you are not. If you aren't ready to conceive, don't push the envelope. You are more fertile now than you will be 3-5 years from now, but your eggs won't turn to dust and blow away when you blow out the candles on your 35th birthday cake.

Sidebar: very few people are ever truly READY to have a baby. You just have to be ready enough, I think. To my 38-year-olds who still want to wait a few more years before trying to have a baby due to career and life, I say don't miss your opportunity. If you feel that pregnancy is a "take it or leave it" endeavor, by all means, wait and see what happens. Pregnancy is still very possible after 40, just less likely. If pregnancy is an absolute life goal, make sure that you don't trade that option for something that in the long run will bring you less fulfillment and possibly more regret.

Egg freezing is an option for those who are financially able and who want to preserve their ability to have babies with their own genetic makeup when they are past the age of reasonable rates of spontaneous conception. In other words, a 40-year-old woman who froze her eggs at 32-years-old can then use her 32-year-old frozen-in-time eggs to conceive via in vitro fertilization (IVF) when her now 40-year-old eggs are too tired to do so. A few facts about egg freezing:

1. This is a cash endeavor. With rare exception (usually cancer-related exceptions), a woman can expect to pay at least $10,000 to have her little genetic jewels preserved.

2. Egg freezing requires multiple injections of hormones to

make a woman prepare to ovulate multiple eggs at one time, instead of her usual single egg. Just before this mass ovulation occurs, the eggs are harvested by needle aspiration and preserved.

3. The optimal age for egg freezing is hard to say, but the younger the better. This is a dichotomous position because the younger a woman is, the better her egg quality will be but the less likely she is to think or know that she may benefit from having frozen eggs in the future. Conversely, the older a woman gets and starts to think, "Hmm, I may need to put these puppies on ice," the less likely those frozen eggs are to result in a successful pregnancy in contrast to her 5-to-10-year-younger self's eggs.

My 40-year-old-eggs comment was not meant to fool anyone into thinking that they cannot conceive past their 30s. My record for the most seasoned woman with a spontaneous (no IVF) conception who I have cared for was 45 years young.

The summary point is that fertility is a continuum that shouldn't be feared from a sudden infertility standpoint, but also shouldn't be taken for granted from a "wait forever before we try" standpoint. If you have been having unprotected vaginal intercourse, you are trying. If you have been trying without conception for 12 months (if you are younger than 35) or 6 months (if older than 35), you should see your gynecologist or infertility specialist. If you have irregular or extremely painful periods, if you or your partner have multiple medical problems (obesity being a common one), or if he has any issues with ejaculation, it is worthwhile to be seen by your physician sooner than the previously mentioned 6-12 months.

Fever

I never truly believed in the back of my momma's hand until I became a momma, and my cheek-on-cheek or back-of-my-hand to forehead game was tested. Normal body temperature is 98.6. There is no doubt that a person can usually feel when another person's temperature is warmer than theirs. Medically, though, there is a number associated with this definition of fever. That number is 100.4. If a digital thermometer says that your body temperature is there or greater, you have a fever. If your temp is 99, or even 100 degrees Fahrenheit, you do not.

This is important, especially if you are pregnant. A fever can signify a severe infection—a kidney infection, mastitis, the flu, ear or sinus infection, or a uterine infection to name a few examples. It is vitally important for you to discuss a fever immediately with your healthcare provider. Acetaminophen (that's Tylenol, but we always had the generic in my house), can decrease your temperature, which can make you feel better. The root cause still should be addressed, though.

In children, the fever story is a little different. When a child is older than three months, the actual number is not nearly as important as how the child behaves. If they are playful and happy, keep them hydrated and watch for worsening of their symptoms. If the child is noticeably feeling bad, it is okay to give them the appropriate amount of Tylenol or ibuprofen, depending on their age and weight, to help them feel better. This point is stressed by the literature—the use of anti-fever meds is ONLY to help the child feel better, rather than to maintain a "normal" temperature. A parent should NOT wake up a sleeping child to give these medications. That's just mean and unnecessary. Fevers should break eventually, so if it lasts five days or more, a doctor visit is warranted.

Healthychildren.org outlined a good summary of when you should call your doctor or consider going to an emergency room. These recommendations are consistent with the American Academy of Pediatrics guidelines. Call your child's doctor right away if your child has a fever and:

• Looks very ill, is unusually drowsy, or is very fussy.

• Has been in a very hot place, such as an overheated car.

• Has other symptoms, such as a stiff neck, severe headache, severe sore throat, severe ear pain, an unexplained rash, or repeated vomiting or diarrhea.

• Has signs of dehydration, such as a dry mouth, sunken soft spot or significantly fewer wet diapers and is not able to take in fluids.

• Has immune system problems, such as sickle cell disease or cancer, or is taking steroids.

• Has had a seizure.

• Is younger than 3 months (12 weeks) and has a temperature of 100.4°F (38.0°C) or higher.

• Fever rises above 104°F (40°C) repeatedly for a child of any age.

Also call your child's doctor if:

• Your child still "acts sick" once his fever is brought down.

• Your child seems to be getting worse.
• The fever persists for more than 24 hours in a child younger than 2 years.
• The fever persists for more than 3 days (72 hours) in a child 2 years of age or older.

Fibroids

These little fibrous balls of excess are the cause of more ultrasound conversations about incidental findings than anything else in my practice. Women with no symptoms but an enlarged uterus noted on exam or pressure and/or heavy bleeding are the all too common recipients of this diagnosis. This one is near and dear to my own heart because my own fibroids were diagnosed when I was but a lowly medical student. I went in for a routine Pap test and Gyne exam. My doctor said that he felt something in my pelvis. Sure enough, it was a 4-centimeter fibroid, about the size of a plum.

Sidebar: have you ever noticed that gynecologists love to describe body parts with fruit or sports? "Her uterus was the size of a grapefruit." "The cyst on her ovary was the size of a softball." It is easier to relate to women with objects rather than just measurements. I just find it kind of funny sometimes when I get to the apricot level and I think, man, I'm going through a lot to find a food to describe this mass.

Double sidebar: My Doc that diagnosed my fibroids was a man. Male OB/GYNs can sometimes feel like a dying breed because women often seem to prefer to see women for their lady issues. No judgment there, but don't discount the fellas, ladies. Male OB/GYNs went through the same training and are just as knowledgeable as we are. The more seasoned guys also have experience on their side. I just had to make that point because one of my partners is a man. He has a strong following of patients, but newbies to the practice sometimes question seeing him. Don't. You won't be sorry.

We re-enter my person fibroid journey when I was pregnant with my eldest son. My dominant fibroid (yes, there were multiples, and no, that is not a thing, but for the purposes of this story, my dominant fibroid was the largest one) was about 10 centimeters— about the size of a softball. Keep in mind, the head of a baby at term is about 10 centimeters from one side to the other. My co-residents used to refer to it as my second baby head because you could even feel it from the outside. After I had my son, it shrank in size dramatically and didn't bother me. I was always on birth control methods that caused me to not have a period, and I believe that helped to stabilize growth.

Fibroids generally don't bother me as the physician and provider, unless they bother the woman who I am caring for. Women with fibroids who don't have heavy bleeding or massive uteruses that are causing uncomfortable bladder or bowel symptoms can keep them as far as I am concerned. As with any rule, there are always exceptions.

The three exceptions to my "But these fibroids aren't bothering me" rule, are scenarios involving desired pregnancy, those where bleeding is so heavy and abundant that anemia is a concern, and the situations where the fibroids are growing rapidly in size. When pregnancy is desired, it is possible to achieve pregnancy when fibroids are in place (guilty as charged), but if a person is deviating from the expected or standard time that it should take to get pregnant, fibroids can be possibly removed to improve the fertility rates. If heavy bleeding is causing anemia, iron supplementation and sometimes removal may need to be discussed. If the size of the uterus is changing rapidly within six months to a year, removal of fibroids may be in order to make sure cancer isn't present.

I will discuss fibroid removal in the section entitled Myomectomy. Isn't this book just full of educational goodness?

4
THE DREADED DR. GOOGLE

G.

Google

All right, I am not trying to get sued. It isn't even worth asking the question of who would win in a legal battle between me and Google. All I am going to say is this: There was this study done by Forbes that looked at the accuracy of online symptom apps in determining the proper diagnoses for patients. Symptoms and Fitbit information were provided to the app. Here were the results:

When doctors in the study were armed with a patient's medical history and symptoms, and then compared with information entered into a symptom checker, doctors arrived at the correct diagnosis 72% of the time, as opposed to 34% for the apps.

Eighty-four percent of the time, doctors provided the correct diagnosis in their top three choices, compared with only 51% for the symptom checkers.

Granted, this study was done with apps rather than Google, but Google has to be worse than this inaccuracy since it doesn't even have any personal data. The point is, typing "What causes x, y and z" into Google is unlikely to get to YOUR diagnosis. Hallelujah (enter the singing angels and the rays of sunlight). No shade on Google (#hellashade) but doctors are better. One tally mark for us.

As I climb down from my soapbox, you may be asking

yourself if I have ever Googled MY OWN symptoms if the diagnosis wasn't clear to me? Yes. I have also been told by Dr. Google that I am about to die within minutes. Just kidding. I feel like I am at a slight advantage because I have at least some discernment as to what is reliable and trustworthy information and what isn't. And I go to the doctor and ask the important questions there. Check out my website gyneco-blogic.com for many more informative health and fun articles if you like a little edu-tainment from time to time.

I wrote a letter to Dr. Google once. It went a little something like this:

Dear Dr. Google,
Stop trying to diagnose my patients' medical problems. It is challenging enough for me to make an accurate diagno-sis after years of training, gathering their full medical history and doing a physical exam. You think that you can do what I do with two words: "What causes..." You are wrong. Stay in your lane.
Sincerely,
Dr. E. W.

Guidelines

I talk a lot about guidelines in my practice. I write a lot about guidelines in this book. I do so because they are what shape my practice as an evidence-based medicine practicing doctor. Imagine that you have a new thing that you want to try. You want to try to eat only carrots for 10 days and see if it will turn your urine orange. If you Google this question and you find one person who said that it works, is that more or less reliable than a study that compared 100 people who tried it and compared their urine to 100 people who ate a non-carrot diet?

If the study was formed in such a way to allow for changes you would see with other food additives, and the people on each side were similar to each other in age and fitness level, etc., that would make the study even more trustworthy and accurate. This is a random example, which I am full of random examples, but the point is that we get medical guidelines and protocols from testing and observing populations over time and determining which is the safest and best course of evaluation and treatment. That is EVIDENCE-based, not GOOGLE CHAT medicine.

The most important thing to know about guidelines is that they are general guides for practice. If a person's specific situation appears to be an outlier, I can change my course of action based on that. A woman with a family history of breast cancer in multiple family members under the age of 50, will not get the same typical guideline-based breast cancer screening as someone without that history. A woman with bleeding with intercourse is not going to get the same every 3-year Pap screening per the typical guidelines. Guidelines guide me, they don't bind me.

How does this apply to you? Well, if you want testing or evaluation that deviates from the standard guidelines, your doctor may or may not agree. If I don't agree with my patient's request, I often still allow them to do the action that they desire, as long as they understand that without a medical indication, the cost of the action may not be covered by insurance. If they understand that, and there is no harm involved, I grant most requests if peace of mind is at stake. Be your own advocate, but work with a doctor who you trust. Those are the keys.

Gyneco-(b)Logic

I couldn't have planned that segue better if I had created the alphabet myself. The Gyneco-(b)Logic was originally started as The Gyneco-Logic on a sleepless night in mid-November 2016. I'm trying to remember what TRAUMATIC, LIFE-CHANGING event had occurred the night prior. Hmmm. My feeling at the exact moment that I began searching my brain for a brand that I could build upon was, "If this just happened, anything can happen, including the start of something big in women's health. [Shrug] Why not start a website?"

I had begun writing my book Angry Wife Happy Wife back in 2012. Angry Wife Happy Wife is a book about marriage. Specifically, it is about remaining happily married for the long haul without trying to stab your husband in the process. If your particular husband is a jerk who is unfaithful or mentally or physically abusive, by all means, get rid of him. But, my book is about that husband who is a good man and a good friend and a good father, but he gets on your DAMN nerves. Though I didn't write in it often, that book was a source of artistic and psychological release for me. I hoped that it would one day become a "thing" that others would benefit from and love as well. I thought that if I started a blog, people would learn who I was and maybe want to read my work later.

The blog has become so much more to me throughout this past year. It was partially the inspiration for this book. In fact, some of my favorite posts have made it into various sections of this book. If you haven't yet, check it out and subscribe at gyneco-blogic.com. The site is full of accurate evidence-based health information and also fun life topics and cool products. You will laugh and learn. I am a fan. You will be, too.

Gynecologist

See Obstetrician. I'll teach you all about gynecology and then some!

H.

Hair

Women generally have two types of problems with their hair. This is aside from the ever-changing style and color choices. Women either complain of having too much hair that is not on their head or too little hair on top of their head. If you think you are losing hair or have thinning hair, that is definitely cause to see an Internal Medicine doctor, also known as an Internist, or a Dermatologist to search for underlying causes. Possible causes range from destructive hairstyles, excessive coloring, or endocrine (hormonal) or autoimmune problems. Don't trust the diagnosis provided to you by the Internet. I don't mind if someone tries skin, hair and nail vitamins, but if the changes are abrupt or dramatic, medical investigation is warranted. Too much hair is a much more common issue. Not too much on top of the head either. We're talking new and more abundant hair on the chin, abdomen, nipple, buttocks, underarm, and many other places. If this subject is Internet searched, hormonal imbalances such as polycystic ovarian syndrome will come up. While hormonal problems can affect hair growth, more commonly, age is a factor in a normal amount of increased hair growth. I'll repeat that one: It is normal for women as we age to grow more hair in unwelcome places. Now it is time to do one of my favorite things—dispel myths:

1. Shaving hair does not make more hair grow. There is nothing about a razor that creates new hair follicles. My very novice understanding of plant, and specifically bush pruning, is that if you trim down dying or overgrown bushes, the growth efforts of the remaining branches will be fuller and more abundant. Razors aren't like that. There is no follicle fertilizer. What a person may notice is that the hair appears darker.

2. The new hair that results from waxing or plucking grows back fine and tapered. This is in contrast to hair that is cut mid-shaft. The full diameter of the remaining hair is what remains, which is wider and broader than the new hair. Take-home message: plucking or waxing will leave less noticeable hair, but shaving won't increase hair quantity.

3. People with coarse hair who are prone to ingrown hairs may need to avoid cutting their unwelcome hair below the skin. I am referring to my ladies who shave the bikini zone and have to answer to ingrown hairs and scars constantly. Those coarse or curly hairs can more easily get trapped under the skin surface when you shave with a razor or when you wax. For those who don't get to the beach regularly, or who just don't care (like me), a better alternative may be to use an electric razor. That way the length and volume of hair can be kept at bay without the individual hairs having to fight their way through the skin. That's what swimsuits with boy shorts are for.

Regarding grays, in short, scientists are beginning to gather clues that stress can hasten the graying process, but there is no scientific evidence demonstrating a clear cause-and-effect relationship. My head would beg to differ. Stress is my middle name sometimes.

I would be remiss if I didn't delve deeper into hair loss related to hair products and styling practices. There are countless articles about the stress, especially on African American heads, caused by chemical and styling techniques. This information is jolting enough to make anyone go natural. Forget being scared straight—you'll be scared curly! I have been fortunate to know Chris-Tia Donaldson, who I met while doing a campaign for breast cancer awareness in 2017. She is a breast cancer survivor and an ambassador for natural hair and skin care. She wrote an amazing book entitled, Thank God I'm Natural: The Ultimate Guide to Caring for and Maintaining Natural Hair. Subsequently, she went on to found TGIN, which is an entire product line of natural skin and hair care products for men and women of all ages and races. I recommend her book and her products to anyone who understands the risks that some unnatural products and ingredients pose to our overall health. If you don't believe me, check out this article from the Environmental Working Group (EWG) about such products. I did not get paid for this endorsement. I just support this cause!

Sources:
http://www.ewg.org/research/big-market-black-cosmetics-less-hazardous-choices-limited#.WeqSaFuPLIU
https://www.scientificamerican.com/article/fact-or-fiction-stress-causes-gray-hair/
https://www.scientificamerican.com/article/fact-or-fiction-if-you-shave-or-wax-your-hair-will-come-back-thicker/

Headaches

There are so many types of headaches and so many causes. I want to highlight a few that have special relevance in the women's health arena: classic, common and menstrual migraines. Classic migraines are those with an aura. An aura is a visual disturbance and other neurological symptoms that appear about 10 to 60 minutes before the actual headache and usually last for no more than an hour. Auras are not painful, but they are notable because a woman who has migraines with aura should ideally not take an estrogen-containing birth control. Migraines with aura are associated with an increased stroke risk for women taking estrogen. Obviously, a woman still releases her own endogenous estrogen, but the additional estrogen added in different types of birth control elevates a woman's risk unnecessarily.

Common migraines are still long and severe headaches, but without aura. Symptoms of a common migraine include moderate to severe pulsating headache pain that occurs without warning and is usually felt on one side of the head. It comes along with nausea, confusion, blurred vision, mood changes, fatigue, and increased sensitivity to light, sound, or smells. Even though stroke risk is less when aura is absent, caution should still be exercised with prescribing estrogen to these ladies. The good news is that there are many estrogen-free birth control options.

Some people have menstrual migraines. That means that for these ladies, the migraine occurs when the period is coming or is present. Basically, old Aunt Flo causes the headache, and thus preventing or skipping Aunt Flo will help eliminate the headaches. For these women, taking birth control pills, with estrogen, continuously is the solution. Skipping the placebo pills, a woman will go straight from one pack to the next fresh medicated tablets. A period is not necessary when hormonal birth control is on board. FYI, it is definitely not okay to skip multiple periods when you are off of any type of hormonal birth control. On the pill, ring, patch, shot, or IUD, periods are totally optional and are not required.

In summary, an occasional headache from time to time is a very common thing. Anyone with recurrent, frequent headaches should consider seeing a doctor. If you are on birth control, see your gynecologist to make sure that your particular birth control is safe with the types of headaches that you have.

Hemorrhoids

Anal blossoms as I like to call them. Actually, I have never called them that. I just thought of that nickname now and will likely never use it again. Hemorrhoids are defined as swollen and inflamed veins in the rectum and anus that cause discomfort and bleeding. Sometimes, these protruding veins come out of the anus, often when a high abdominal pressure situation is in place, like pregnancy. Some causes are chronic constipation, which can lead to frequent bearing down and pushing, and pregnancy and delivery. Yes, the act of pushing can also make hemorrhoids worse. So what's wrong with this grape bunch protruding from your anus? Well, hemorrhoids can bleed, but they can also hurt, BADLY. Thrombosed, or clotted, hemorrhoids can cause pain that can make it hard to sit, walk or just live a normal life. These puppies send women to the ER when they are extremely bad. What can be done? Steroid cream can decrease the inflammation that causes the intense pain. Numbing spray or ointment can take some of the sensation away. They cannot be surgically removed during pregnancy, and the word on the street is that surgical removal is one of the most painful surgeries to recover from.

What is the good news? They are usually at their worst when a woman is pregnant. Then they improve during and after the postpartum period. Will they ever go away spontaneously? Most likely not without surgical intervention, but unless they are bleeding or painful, they can just stay. That is unless you are one of those anal bleaching types who is concerned about the external appearance of your anus. My ass could care less. #punlife.

History and Physical

I am not going to belabor the point too much. I just ranted a little bit ago about the dangers of Dr. Google. I have to highlight one last important factor when we talk about why an in-person human doctor is better than Google. Three letters: HNP. Actually, it is H&P, which stands for history and physical. It is the first thing taught in the clinical portion of medical school and it is how we physicians can help draw a conclusion about what is wrong with you, if anything. The components are the History of Present Illness, or HPI, the Review of Systems, the Past Medical History, Past Surgical History, Family History, Medication List, Social History, and the Physical Exam. I have a relevant point in sharing this information. Bear with me.

The HPI is where we ask when your symptoms started, how long they have been occurring, how severe they are, what makes them better or worse. All of these questions serve as puzzle pieces leading toward the diagnosis. If I ask you, how long, please don't say, "A while." What is a while? A day? A week? A year? When I feel like a dentist (pulling teeth) to get chronologic information from ladies, I will often say "Were you having this issue last year this time? What about last month?" Use your electronic devices to help. Plug symptoms into your phone notepad or calendar. Download a period tracker app, a free one, before you go see your Gyne and complain about irregular bleeding. If you can remember how often and how long with details, great. If not, write that stuff in a paper notebook if you have to. I can't put this puzzle together if a lot of the pieces are blurry or blank.

Another H&P roadblock that often makes us doctors internally shake our heads is the family history. What has happened to your family members, especially close relatives, is relevant when it comes to what could be happening to you. It is important even if you think that their disease was self-inflicted. A good example of this is when people tell me that a family member had diabetes, "but it was because they were overweight." Even if that were true, it still counts toward your risk. There are plenty of people who are not overweight who can still develop diabetes if their genetics predispose them. Conversely, there are plenty of people who are overweight who will not develop "the sugar" as the old folk call it. It all counts. If your family is the type that doesn't like to talk about medical problems, assure your family members that knowing what to be on the lookout for can actually lower your risk of developing certain diseases.

Knowing your family history can lower your risk of developing diseases in many ways. A great scenario to support this point is colon cancer prevention. Colonoscopies are generally recommended to start at the age of 50 for most people, 45 for African Americans. If you know of a first-degree relative, like a sibling or parent, who developed precancerous colon polyps or colon cancer, your screening should begin 10 years before that person was found to have their first polyp. For example, if my dad had polyps when he was 50, I should have my first colonoscopy at age 40. That way if anything were starting to grow earlier than normal for me, I can make sure that it is removed and won't turn into cancer over time.

Talk to your family about your medical diagnoses and encourage your family members to do the same with you. If seeing the train coming in the distance will decrease the chances that I am in the railroad crossing by the time it arrives, that's a win. By the way, if you haven't noticed by now, I am the queen of random analogies.

Human Papillomavirus

HPV is a virus that is so commonly misunderstood. First of

all, it is everywhere. From the Center for Disease Control: Human Papillomavirus (HPV) is the most common sexually transmitted infection in the United States. Over 40 distinct HPV types can infect the genital tract. Although most infections are asymptomatic and appear to resolve spontaneously within a few years, prevalence of genital infection with any HPV type was 42.5% among United States adults aged 18–59 years during 2013–2014. Persistent infection with some HPV types can cause cancer and genital warts. HPV types 16 and 18 account for approximately 66% of cervical cancers in the United States, and approximately 25% of low-grade and 50% of high-grade cervical intraepithelial lesions, or dysplasia. HPV types 6 and 11 are responsible for approximately 90% of genital warts.
Reference: https://www.cdc.gov/std/stats16/other.htm#hpv

CDC, I couldn't have said it better myself. Some points of clarification: A person doesn't always know if they have HPV. With the exception of the types that cause warts, the virus can live on the skin and be spread through contact without any symptoms. Even the types that cause warts don't always cause warts right away and can do this to varying degrees. Genital warts can be mistaken for skin tags and other lesions as well. See my section on Things, as in Things on your Thing, for more about the confusion revolving around genital lesions and how to try to know what is what.

HPV prevention can come from decreasing exposure and getting vaccinated. To decrease exposure, limiting the number of sexual partners is the best way to prevent transmission. Condoms help to limit transmission but aren't a perfect solution because the virus can be present on areas of the skin not covered by condoms. The Human Papillomavirus 9-valent Vaccine is a vaccine that tries to prevent 9 strains of HPV from being contracted. Remember, there are over 40 strains of HPV, so it is not perfect. There is some cross-protection provided by being vaccinated by some strains that should at least decrease your risk of contracting others. Plus, the nine strains present in the vaccine are known to be the more aggressive and common strains.

The bottom line is that HPV is everywhere. Decreasing your exposure via limiting sexual contact is the best form of prevention. After that, the vaccine is helpful, but not fool proof. A person should still get their Pap tests as indicated (see the section on Pap) and be evaluated for any new or changing skin lesions in areas of sexual contact, or any area on the body for that matter, even if HPV isn't suspected.

Hymen

A woman's natural chastity belt. (Bwah ha ha, yeah, right.) The hymen stops just about as much sex as, as, as something that doesn't stop sex. Why would I liken it to a chastity belt then? Because the times when I encounter a hymen professionally, it is usually in the setting of a vagina that is so constricted by a very narrow hymen, the woman cannot have sex, and sometimes cannot even use tampons.

There are many anatomical features that can cause a vagina to be "dysfunctional" for penetrative intercourse. An imperforate, or closed, hymen is one of the possible diagnoses. Another is a transverse vaginal septum—essentially a fleshy wall inside of the vagina. Another big one is a genetic abnormality that causes a sex chromosome misfire during embryologic development and leaves a "woman" with NO vagina.

What did she just say?

Yes, there are a number of genetic disorders that can occur during the development of the uterus (the womb for my "womb" term lovers) that can lead to a baby being born with ambiguous genitalia, not clearly boy or girl parts. There is a syndrome that causes a person to look externally like a girl but to have testes (testicles inside of the abdomen), a Y chromosome (46 XY to be exact) that will lead to a very short vagina and no uterus. This is called androgen insensitivity. A longstanding rumor among many in Hollywood is that Jamie Lee Curtis has this syndrome. This rumor was never substantiated, and I prefer to mind my own business. I bring this up because the diagnosis isn't always clear. There are a few tactics that I can use to determine if someone who can't use her vagina for anything fun has an imperforate hymen or some other syndrome.

First, if an adult woman has external features to reflect her believed sex—breasts, underarm and pubic hair—that's a good sign that her sex genes are XX. Secondly, if she has a period every month, that is a good sign that she has female internal organs. If she is an adolescent with cyclic, monthly abdominal pain without bleeding, this could be a sign of a transverse vaginal septum or completely occluded hymen. It is possible that she is bleeding every month, but the blood just can't get out of the vaginal canal. Ultrasound or MRI can be used to investigate this suspicion. If she has a period every month with nothing more than light cramps, the blood is likely escaping out of a small hole in the hymen that is often too small to admit even a tampon.

In these situations, I usually try to perform an exam in the office, but more often we end up needing to go to the operating room for an exam under anesthesia due to discomfort.

Once in the operating room, an anesthesiologist can put her to sleep, and I can examine the woman without discomfort. It is often useful for the woman to be on her period during this exam so that I can see where the blood is emerging from. Then I can attempt to insert a small 3-millimeter scope into the vagina to look for the cervix and confirm that we are where I think we are. Once the location is confirmed, I can incise and open the hymen and voila! We've OPENED UP a whole new world of possibilities. #punlife

What is the take-home message here? If a woman has never used a tampon or had sex because of difficulty, pain or discomfort, it is worth checking in with a Gyne who can evaluate her and make sure that anatomically everything is in working order. If standard anatomy can be confirmed, then physical therapy or psychotherapy may be of assistance. If anatomy cannot be confirmed during an awake exam, imaging and/or sedation with anesthesia are appropriate next steps. Let's CLOSE UP this topic. #Canthelpit

Hysterectomy

Hysterectomy is defined as the removal of the uterus (womb if you NEED me to say that. This is the last time though.) Oopherectomy is the removal of the ovaries. There are not only many ways to perform this surgery, but there are many decisions to be made about which organs can and should be removed during the surgery.

There was a day when just about everyone had a hysterectomy. You have allergies? Hyst. You have heel spurs? Hyst. You're crazy? Hyst. No jokes on that one. The etymology of the term hyster—which is the prefix to describe the uterus comes from the Latin term hystericus, which is hysteria in English. They literally used to believe that when women went psycho, it was because of their uterus and if that were removed, she wouldn't be crazy anymore. If you think I'm crazy now, check on me after your rudimentary, ancient medical ass removes my uterus without sterile technique or even anesthesia in most cases. The origins of modern medicine, especially as it relates to women and ESPECIALLY women of color are truly sickening. If you question how I felt from my intro, may I add, EFF YOU J. Marion Sims (I don't curse but If I did…). They called him the Father of Gynecology. Well, J., for all of the atrocities you did to African American women to make your pivotal discoveries, you can kiss the Father of MY ASS! I know that doesn't make any sense, but the sentiment stands.

Whew, now that that rant is over…these days, a lot of the problems that led women like my mom to have a hysterectomy can be remedied in other ways. We have medication and minimally invasive procedures that help women control bleeding, pain and growth of fibroids, etc. Sometimes a hysterectomy is still needed, but far less frequently than even 20 years ago.

If you do need that uterus removed, the first question to ask and answer is what needs to go? Are we removing just the uterus? The uterus and ovaries and tubes (bilateral salpingo-oopherectomy)? The cervix too? If there has been a significant history of cervical dysplasia—which means precancerous changes on the cervix—the cervix should absolutely be removed. Other than that, there are pros and cons to removal of the cervix which don't make it an obvious decision one way or another. Since there is little evidence of any benefit of leaving the cervix within a woman's body, if it is surgically possible without too much risk, I usually recommend removing it. There is almost no reliable evidence that keeping the cervix benefits the woman. It doesn't prevent prolapse, or falling of the vagina or bladder, and it doesn't add to the enjoyment of sex in any meaningful way. Truly! This was studied. Don't ask me how researchers did that study, exactly, but we have data.

Whether the ovaries stay or go is mainly dependent on the woman's age and personal or family history of ovarian issues, including endometriosis and cancer. The tubes almost always should go as a cancer risk reduction measure. More on that in the Tubes section. Ultimately, these decisions are best made between a woman and her operating doctor, not Google, or even this book.

How are we going to get this uterus out? It can be removed via laparotomy, laparoscopy, robotic surgery or vaginally. Laparotomy means either a horizontal (like a C-section) or vertical abdominal incision. This is often best for large bulky, fibroid ridden uteruses, primarily because of size alone. Laparoscopic and robotic surgeries are usually better for smaller uteruses with concern for pre-cancer (worrisome atypia) or endometrial (uterine) cancer. This uterus is often dissected away from the body along with other possibly affected organs and structures like lymph nodes, using little robotic arms that are inserted through numerous small 1-2 cm incisions in the abdomen. While the operative time is often longer than with an open case (laparotomy), the recovery is usually faster and less intense from a pain standpoint. In the hand of someone who does these surgeries frequently, operating times are often much lower and uteruses of slightly larger sizes can sometimes be tackled.

A vaginal hysterectomy is by far the fastest and easiest to recover from, but not every uterus can come through the vagina, and not every vagina will permit the descent and removal of a uterus. Did I just say the same thing twice? No. To clarify, a super large bulky uterus can rarely be removed safely through the vagina, even a "larger" vagina that has delivered multiple babies. Conversely, even a small, normal sized uterus can sometimes not be removed safely through a very narrow, tight, long vagina.

There is definitely surgical skill involved in reducing the risk of complications in vaginal surgery. You may be thinking, "Isn't there skill required for any surgery?" Yes, but some surgeries are more technically challenging than others. Some require real-time troubleshooting that may not be easy for every OB/GYN. I have been fortunate to operate with seasoned doctors who have taught me more amazing surgical techniques even after my training completed. Because of this, I feel very confident performing vaginal hysterectomies when appropriate, but some may not. It is up to the skill and comfort of the surgeon, as well as the anatomy of the woman, to determine if a vaginal hysterectomy is even an option at all.

Let this and other procedural sections of this book serve to increase your understanding about the procedures themselves, but know that your individual treatment plan is between you and your doctor, not me, unless I am your doctor (aww, thanks for buying my book! Bring it to your next appointment and I'll sign it if you want! I'm touched—no pun intended). Also, never be afraid to get a second opinion if you either don't understand or don't agree with a treatment plan. I would always prefer that a person explore all of their options if they are concerned. I don't want you to feel like you have unanswered questions, and I definitely don't want you to be dissatisfied with your care, any more than you want to be.

Hysteroscopy

This is a minimally invasive procedure that is used to remove anything necessary from the inside of the uterus. It is a scope or camera that fits through the vagina and cervix to look in the uterus and can be used to remove polyps, fibroids, perform a targeted biopsy, perform a tubal ligation via occlusion of the tubes from the inside, and even rarely, remove a foreign body like an IUD whose strings are unable to be found (that is RARE y'all. IUDs are great).

Hysteroscopy is one of the procedures that make hysterectomies less common. Under light anesthesia, so many causes of heavy or irregular bleeding can be removed. This long cylinder-like instrument, the width of an old-school Bic pen can be passed into the vagina, through the cervix, and into the uterus. The uterus can be examined and abnormal findings can often be removed.

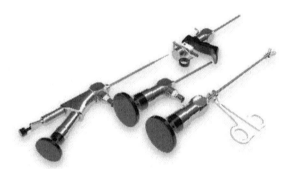

Hysteroscopy can be done using sleeping sedation or local anesthesia while awake in the office. The type of anesthesia that I request is dependent on what I plan to do. The more extensive the surgery, the more uncomfortable I would expect the patient to be. If it is a minor procedure, then having an awake patient who is anesthetized (numbed) with local lidocaine may be just enough. This is very similar to when a dentist numbs a part of your mouth with injected lidocaine prior to dental work. The same thing can be done with the cervix and uterus. My patient's anxiety level also plays a role. If she passes out during the preoperative consultation, this may not be the woman that I want to stay awake during surgery.

What hysteroscopy cannot do well is evaluate if the tubes

are opened. It can also not be used to evaluate the ovaries, because as you can see, the hysteroscopic view is of the inside of the uterus. The ovaries and the rest of the pelvis are on the outside of the uterus. Endometrial ablation is a procedure that can be done using hysteroscopy to control heavy uterine bleeding. Initially, the tissue lining of the uterus, or the endometrium, must be evaluated for any signs of pre-cancer or cancer. This can be done with an in-office biopsy or with a D&C in the operating room, which stands for dilation and curettage. Dilation is the manual opening of the cervix. Curettage means scraping. Both an endometrial biopsy and a D&C are two methods to sample the tissue in the uterus and make sure that it is normal and you are safe, even if it is misbehaving and making you bleed too much or at sucky times.

Hormone levels should also be checked. A thyroid abnormality can cause abnormal bleeding, for example. A complete blood count (CBC), and specifically the hemoglobin, should be checked. If that level is low, that is called anemia. Anemia can be managed with either iron supplementation to help you make more blood or by decreasing the amount of blood loss. Hysteroscopic ablation can often help with the latter.

Three downsides to know about endometrial ablations are as follows: (1) The effects aren't always permanent. If you are 45, you have a better chance of this procedure controlling your bleeding through menopause than if you are 35 years old. (2) After having an ablation, the uterus may be more difficult to evaluate for new abnormalities later in life. This is due to the scarring that an ablation creates. (3) Pregnancy is strongly discouraged after an ablation. It is important to realize that fertility rates decrease post-ablation, but a woman who is still ovulating can still conceive even in an ablated uterus, but with a high likelihood for complications. Birth control is recommended.

The take-home message: If your doctor offers you a hysteroscopy to treat your bleeding abnormality, make sure that you are evaluated thoroughly and then consider trying it. Hysteroscopy is a minimally invasive procedure and is often a pretty good idea. Just make sure, as always, that you agree with what is being evaluated, how you are being treated, and that you understand the chances of success and the risks.

I.

Illicit Drugs

Marijuana to be specific. This is a book about popcorn (not really), which is a common snack to munch on. I digress. I have never smoked, eaten, or inserted marijuana anywhere in or around my body. I do, however, know what it smells like. What person who has been to college, or lived at all, doesn't. I am including this little blurb because it has come up in the literature as a treatment for the symptoms associated with endometriosis and pelvic pain. This is not surprising since it is useful for managing symptoms associated with cancer and chemotherapy. I wanted to give a quick shout out to the evidence though.

A PubMed search revealed a number of scholarly articles from as long ago as 2010. One stated the following, "The endocannabinoid system contributes to mechanisms underlying both the peripheral innervation of the abnormal growths and the pain associated with endometriosis, thereby providing a novel approach for the development of badly-needed new treatments."

Reference: Dmitrieva N, Nagabukuro H, Resuehr D, et al. Endocannabinoid involvement in endometriosis. Pain. 2010;151(3):703-710. doi:10.1016/j.pain.2010.08.037.

More research and a change in the laws of the state of Illinois will be needed before I expand on this topic any further in this book. Until then, do you.

Incontinence

Ahhh incontinence. One of my favorite things…to treat I mean. I like it because I like things that I have a good chance of successfully fixing. When a woman can be brought from laughing golden sprinkles to holding her urine like a big kid, that is truly fulfilling. Do I have a 100% cure rate? No, but a woman could possibly have a 0% cure rate if she never talks to someone about it or seeks help. Something is better than nothing.

Urinary incontinence is the involuntary loss of urine. It can occur as a result of different activities or actions and can be caused by a variety of events. A common misconception is that if a woman can avoid a vaginal delivery, she will save herself from incontinence in the future. Nice try, but that's not true. Pregnancy alone has been shown to increase a woman's risk for developing incontinence over time, even if she delivers via cesarean section or if she vaginally delivers a small baby. Now a severe tear can put a damper on a woman's pelvic floor muscle control, but these are not the only women who are plagued by this annoying and embarrassing problem.

Urinary incontinence is divided into types—two of the most common being Stress and Urge. If you remember the "Gotta go, gotta go, gotta go right now!" commercials, those were for a medication that treats the urgent sensation to urinate that would make you push a grandmother and her toddler grandchild out of line in the bathroom. Stress incontinence is the type that catches women off guard with a sneeze, cough, run or laugh. You think that your co-worker doesn't think any of your jokes are funny, but really she just doesn't want to wet herself laughing at your terrible jokes.

There are various levels of evaluation and treatment for urinary incontinence. Fecal and flatus (gas) incontinence are also symptoms that should be evaluated by a physician. A woman can start to treat minor symptoms of urinary incontinence with Kegel, exercises, which I will tackle in the K section. If symptoms persist, don't just deal with it, get evaluated. I mentioned that I like treating this because it IS often something that I can help improve.

Infertility

I touched on this topic in the Fertility section, but let's delve a little deeper into the definition and initial workup of infertility. A doc who I trained underused to say, "Women spend half of their reproductive years trying to not get pregnant and the other half trying to." Deep. I have never personally experienced this challenge, but I have seen firsthand how frustrating and all-consuming it can be for some. Like in many aspects of medicine, there are some things that we can control, and some that we can't. There are steps, though, to help women navigate the evaluation process.

You know that I love my definitions. Infertility is defined as the inability to conceive after a year of unprotected penile-vaginal intercourse for women under the age of 35, or after six months for any woman 35 years old or older. The fact that this definition leaves out the male age is just a testament to the fact that men can be, not that they always are, fertile until they are senior citizens. I'm not just talking about Isaac in the Bible. I'm talking about (courtesy of Babble.com) Robert DeNiro (68), Steve Martin (67), Nick Nolte (66), Michael Douglas (58), Hugh Hefner (66), Julio Iglesias (63), Clint Eastwood (66), and Michael Jordan (50) to name a few celebrity examples.

Did I have to specify penile-vaginal intercourse? Well, my senior partner told me a story of a couple who came to him for evaluation of infertility. They were both virgins. (Yes, I told this story earlier in the book, but for those skipping around, it is a good story that bears repeating.) When they got married, they found themselves not being able to get pregnant. They didn't know until he, a seasoned gynecologist, gathered enough information to discover they had been having anal intercourse the whole time. What a revelation. There are no eggs back there.

Infertility is different from recurrent pregnancy loss, which still results in the lack of a baby, but for a different reason. A woman who can conceive, but repeatedly loses the baby, more than twice by definition, garners the diagnosis of recurrent pregnancy loss. While one miscarriage sucks, really sucks, it is not defining. It does not set a woman on a trajectory of always losing a baby. One miscarriage can happen to anyone once, or even twice. There is a rule in medicine that anything that happens to a person once is more likely to happen to them again. More than likely, though, one miscarriage still falls into the realm of a spontaneous and unexplained occurrence that is unlikely to happen again.

The most likely reason for a miscarriage is a spontaneous chromosomal abnormality. This can occur as a result of the presence of an egg or a sperm containing the wrong number of chromosomes. Contrary to what some believe, we are not perfect, and neither are all of our gametes (i.e. every egg or every sperm). Enter my Bachelor's Degree in Biology.

As humans, we each should have 46 chromosomes in every cell in our bodies. When it is time to conceive and create another human, the building blocks for this are an egg and sperm, which are both called gametes. Before a gamete is primed and ready to fertilize or be fertilized, the precursor cells have to divide their original 46 chromosomes down to 23. That way, each gamete brings 23 chromosomes to the fertilization party, which add together to give the new human 46 chromosomes of their own. If that split doesn't happen just right, the gametes can be left with 24 and 22 chromosomes rather than 23 and 23. Sometimes a gamete can even have partial chromosomes. When the egg and sperm then unite, if a 23-chromosome sperm unites with a 24-chromosome egg, that 47-chromosome zygote (early, early baby) may not survive, or it may form a person who is abnormal genetically. Down syndrome is an example where there are three of a particular chromosome rather than two. That's why it is called TRIsomy 21—three copies of chromosome #21, totaling 47 chromosomes rather than 46. Many don't survive, or if they do, they often have health and developmental challenges.

Genetic abnormalities can lead to miscarriage or infertility. Other possible causes and risk factors for infertility include abnormal sperm quantity and quality (apart from the chromosome portion), blocked fallopian tubes, abnormal uterine cavity if fibroids or polyps are present, endometriosis, hormonal abnormalities and other medical problems like high blood pressure and diabetes. If you have been having unprotected penile-vaginal intercourse for more than the previously mentioned times without a pregnancy, talk to your gynecologist about what can be done next to move you closer to a safe and healthy pregnancy.

Itching

See Vaginitis. I know you are itching to read about this subject.

IUD

See the Contraception topic. I'm out of witty puns at this exact moment. Stay around though.

5
FIVE GOLDEN GYNECOLOGISTS
OR ONE

J.

Jaundice

All three of my children developed jaundice shortly after birth. They all even had to stay in the hospital longer than normal admission because of it. Jaundice is defined as an excess accumulation of bilirubin in the blood. This can occur when an adult is in liver failure or has severe hepatitis, but in my newborns, it was caused by a mild blood type incompatibility which led to an excess blood product break down, resulting in increased blood levels of bilirubin. The only way that babies can get rid of the excess is by skin exposure to ultraviolet light and through bowel movements. If they don't get rid of the bilirubin fast enough, it can cause a toxicity in the brain that can lead to brain damage.

Medical history moment: Before jaundice was well understood, it was a known finding that babies in the nursery who were closer to the window did better than babies who were away from the windows. Unbeknownst to the early observers, the sunlight was able to help some of the babies eliminate this extra blood breakdown byproduct. Now, I pushed all three of my newborn babies to the windows of my postpartum rooms and they ALL still ended up under the bili lights. Thank you, modern technology. My progeny may not have made it through back in the day before the era of modern science.

Jejunum

Did you know that different parts of the small bowel, also known as small intestines, have different names? The jejunum is the portion of the small bowel where most of your nutrients are absorbed. The duodenum and the ileum are the other parts of the small bowel. There are a lot of small bowel diseases, but I don't want to talk about those in this book. By "don't want to," I also mean "can't because I don't know." I'll leave topics about the intestines and absorption for my esteemed Gastroenterology specialist husband. Dr. Edwin McDonald, IV, founder of TheDocsKitchen.com. The end.

K.

Kegel Exercises

You know that you are both old AND wise when a sneeze comes with an automatic Kegel. It shows forethought and prevention of an accident that you used to think only happened to potty-training toddlers. Alas, if you have been through my section on incontinence, you know that the bladder does not have eyes or ears. It does not always know when you are on the toilet versus when you are sitting at your desk, standing in line at the grocery store, or watching a movie that is just getting to the good part. If your pelvic muscles tend to relax at the most inopportune time, you may need to call in reinforcements in that pelvic floor.

A Kegel exercise is a voluntary contraction of the muscles of the pelvic floor. These are the same muscles used to hold urine, hold in gas, and push out bowel movements or babies (or both at the same time in some cases). A person, in theory, should be able to stop their urine midstream by contracting these muscles. I say "in theory" because that is not a very comfortable action to perform and is often an unnecessary test of the strength of the pelvic floor. A

Kegel is not an abdominal muscle work out. Your face does not have to move to perform a Kegel exercise. If I coach a woman to isolate these muscles, I make sure her abs are relaxed and that she is not using her thighs either.

I once saw a woman holding a surfboard with her vagina. She was posting on some news or social media platform and had a series of pictures of her holding various heavy items from a string emerging from beneath the leg hole in her shorts. This woman had an ovule of some sort attached to a string, attached to items weighing more than many items I would want to hold with an outstretched arm, let alone with my vagina. Why would she do such a thing? She claimed that having rock-hard Kegels (that doesn't even look right on paper) helped her have stronger orgasms and not leak urine. I can support her desire to stay dry, but an orgasm from a vagina strong enough to hold a surfboard sounds like it would do more damage than good to the other partner. The anticipation alone seems like it would make a man nervously limp. If you haven't already guessed, I don't recommend a woman hold anything in her vagina for any purpose. Having strong Kegel muscles can, however, save a woman wet-clothing embarrassment.

So what is the best way to perform Kegel exercises? I recommend that my patients perform ten 2-3 second contractions of the pelvic floor at least twice daily. I also think it helps to have triggers to remember to do them. A reminder in your phone, a radio morning show, or a meeting at work can all be times and places triggering your recollection of the need for this much needed regular exercise. My best trigger is while I am coaching one of my patients to push out a baby. While I am counting to ten during each of her intense pushes, I am counting out my own Kegel session so that nothing falls out of my own vagina without my consent.

Check out my YouTube channel, keyword DrEveryWoman, if you haven't already seen me perform SWV, Weak about bladder trials and tribulations. Make sure that your bladder is trained before you listen in public though. It may challenge your dryness.

Kidneys

Introducing urinary tract infections (UTIs). Actually, not to fake you out, but we will tackle recurrent UTIs and ways to recognize and prevent them in the UTI section. I want to discuss kidney infections and kidney stones here though because they are a different beast. UTIs are a nuisance. Kidney infections are dangerous. Let's go back to anatomy. A woman urinates out of the urethra, which is located between the opening of the vagina and the clitoris. If we go due north within the urethra (Magic School Bus style), we run straight into the urine reservoir known as the bladder. The road then splits into two tubes called the ureters. They are on the left and the right behind the abdominal cavity, closer to the back. These ureters travel up to the kidneys. Though we took this anatomic journey northward, the urine actually flows straight down to the dirty south. Our blood flows through and is "cleaned" by the kidneys, and all of the bi-products and extras, including excess water, are formed into urine by the kidneys. Even though the kidneys "clean" the blood, urine is not dirty with bacteria. It is actually sterile (bacteria-free). Bacteria is all over the vaginal area though.

The vagina and anus are full of an abundance of bacteria. If any of that bacteria is able to multiply and ascend into the urethra, through the bladder, up the ureters and make its way to the kidneys, that infection is known as pyelonephritis. It causes fevers, back pain, and can become a serious infection requiring hospitalization. This is important because if a urinary tract infection is improperly or incompletely treated, a person could be susceptible to serious disease and organ damage. Seeing a healthcare provider for proper treatment if a kidney infection is suspected is very important.

Not every back pain is a kidney infection. Back pain can be musculoskeletal pain. It could be a kidney stone, which can be extremely painful. Women can be more susceptible to kidney stones if they are dehydrated, are obese and have specific medical problems or dietary limitations. If you have a kidney stone frequent flier card, you should discuss prevention with your doctor.

Let's talk about dialysis for a second. So many people in my community have diabetes. Severe stages of this disease can lead to kidney damage. Dialysis is required when a person has such severe renal (kidney) disease that they can't "clean" their own blood. The machine mixes a solution with the blood to get out all of the unwanted waste and regulates the minerals and metabolites in the blood. The only way that a person with end-stage renal disease can free themselves from having this done every few days is to get a kidney transplant. #beadonor #trynottodiethough #youonlyneedonekidney.

K-Y Jelly

I'll save this topic for the lubrication section, unless K-Y wants to cut me a separate check. Get at me K-Y.

Kyphosis

That hunchback that you always wondered about in the elderly woman who you knew? That's Kyphosis. No need to get too preoccupied with medical terminology, but you should know what it is because there are ways to prevent it. Kyphosis often occurs as a result of multiple vertebral fractures. These fractures over time cause the spinal spaces to narrow and basically collapse on one another. It's like an accordion being crushed by body weight. Did you ever wonder why certain people's grandmothers seem so short even if they didn't look like the hunchback of Notre Dame? The same reasons apply. This hunching of the upper back or loss of height can also be caused by the soft cushiony disks between the boney vertebrae breaking down. It's like that old mattress that needs to be replaced and sinks down in the center. It's a good thing that our backs take way longer than seven years to break down. Unfortunately, you can't just hit up a Mattress Firm store for new vertebral discs on Memorial Day.

There are other causes for kyphosis other than vertebral compression fractures and degenerating discs, but as you probably have noticed so far, I like to focus my topics on the biggest players. If you want the rare red-herring, that's what Google is for. I take a lot of cheap shots at Google, but that's because it messes with my patients and friends who are searching for answers. It's like The Rock said in Central Intelligence, "I don't like bullies!"

Preventing vertebral compression fractures starts with understanding why they happen. Osteoporosis is a major cause for a person's bones to not be strong enough to support their body weight into old age. It is not just a disease for frail white women either. Anyone with lower body weight and a low calcium diet can be at risk because bone strength often corresponds to the amount of work that is demanded of the bone. Let me try that one again: If bones have to bear a lot of weight or endure a lot of weight bearing exercise, they respond by staying stronger (your body builds more bone). This is one situation where people of higher body weight actually are winning. Before you get too excited, remember that being overweight or obese can actually over-stress the joints and spine and increase the risk for disc herniation and nerve impingement, which can cause pain.

Stay tuned for more ways to tackle and combat low bone mass and osteoporosis in the Osteoporosis section. As for those discs, not smoking, low impact exercise like walking, swimming and yoga, and a healthy diet can help the spine stay as healthy as possible as our life seasons change.

L.

Labia

What are those? Take your chapter-skipping self back up to the Anatomy section. Look for and read the section about the vulva. Thank you.

If you know what they are but are unsure if yours are normal, know this: There are so many labial shapes and sizes, you don't even know. There is an art piece called The Great Wall of Vagina, by a UK sculptor Jamie McCartney. This dude (yes, I said dude) made plaster casts of 400 vulvas from ages 18-76. We are talking 10 columns of 40 vaginas each. If you think I'm lying, take it to Google. The Huffington Post did a whole story about it. It's fascinating. Not enough for me to have any replicas in my home or office, but I still appreciate the artistic dedication of spending five years casting and making plaster replicas of 400 vaginas. I just hope he used new plaster each time. No double dipping, please.

Women can compare many things between themselves and other ladies, but the vagina/vulva isn't an area often compared. I am not advocating for such comparisons, but I do like this particular piece of art because it highlights the fact that women can be so different and still each be normal. I have done surgeries in the past to decrease the length of the labia because they were uncomfortable physically. Maybe they were irritating in intimate moments or sore after long bike rides. When I encounter someone who wants their labia altered because she thinks that they look abnormal, I carefully challenge her to understand that normal is not one specific appearance. The Great Wall of Vagina displays our differences as unique and special.

Moving on…

Labor and Delivery

This one is going to be a doozy. I could write a whole book about this subject, but I am going to focus on three topics:

- Why did I deliver my own three babies at a hospital?
- What are the stages of labor?
- What are the most important things for a man to do while the mother of his child is pregnant or in labor?

I am not trying to mess with anyone who wants to deliver their baby at home. There are two types of women who I try not to confront directly: Women who want homebirths and women who breastfeed their kids until they are teenagers. I have always said that a term baby cannot come out too fast. "Term" as it relates to the age of a pregnancy means that the baby is old enough to not be considered premature or too young to be delivered. Short of the trauma to a woman's carpet or car upholstery, generally speaking, a term baby who just decides to come out of their momma's vagina like a slip and slide is going to be just fine. Wrap that baby up, rub its feet to make it cry, and wait for the paramedics.

I don't worry about those babies. The babies that I worry about are the ones who get stuck, whether in the uterus because the cervix never reaches 10 centimeters, or in the vagina as a woman pushes and pushes, but that baby just won't come out. This is where my fear of homebirths comes in. It's not the easy deliveries, but the ones that have complications which challenge the health of the mom and baby. Often the amount of time that I as the doctor have to react to signs of trouble is brief. If you aren't even in a hospital, that elapsed time increases, raising the odds of mom and baby experiencing longstanding health issues and life-threatening complications.

Then, if that baby comes out, whether after resisting eviction or through the aforementioned slip and slide, the most dangerous thing for a woman in the US during the birthing process is the threat of hemorrhage in the postpartum period. Blood loss during childbirth is normal and expected, but if it is too excessive, a woman can undergo serious injury or death. I personally had the pleasure of having one of my kids delivered using vacuum and forceps, one child while I had preeclampsia, and one child while I had cholestasis of pregnancy, all of which are serious conditions unable to be managed at home. I didn't know that any of those things were going to happen to me. If I were oblivious to the goings-on in my body, I may not have three happy healthy children to show for it. Wearing a seatbelt might not prevent a car accident, but it can save you if the unexpected happens. This is why I had my babies at a hospital.

The stages of labor are like the ABCs for me as an OB/GYN. I marvel when a patient asks me a question about what happens first and next. It sounds like this: "So, there's A, then B. Then what's after that?" I realize though, that the world I live in isn't one that is common to everyone. That is why I wrote this book: to bring you all into the Chronicles of OB/GYNia. Am I like the lion? I want that wardrobe though.

Stage 1 consists of the latent and active phases of labor.

Stage 2 is the pushing stage.

Stage 3 is the stage that occurs between the delivery of the baby and the delivery of the placenta.

If you think your water has broken before going into labor, call your doctor and head to the hospital. A "dry birth" is not a thing. The bag of water is full of fluid that comes from the placenta and from baby urine. Both are continually produced. Even women whose bag of water breaks weeks before they are due are sometimes able to stay pregnant with fluid in the uterus for days or weeks because more fluid is constantly being made. The term "dry birth" makes my vagina uncomfortable, and I'm not even pregnant. Rest assured, ladies, even with very little fluid, pregnant vaginas are generally anything but dry.

Men, your role, while this glorious woman with a crown around her midsection is having a baby, is to support her, save her from herself, and love that baby. This is a challenging place to be. It is like trying to protect a captive wild animal from hurting herself in a cage. If you get in that cage with her, she might just maul you to death. Shooting a pregnant woman with a tranquilizer gun isn't exactly P.C. Those hormones are raging and she may be a peaceful flower or a venomous beast. I use that term with all affection since I have sported some fangs in my day, or so I'm told. (He didn't use those exact words though because I would have cut him.)

Ladies, it's time to pass the book to the dad-to-be, present or future.

Don't worry, guy. I won't keep you long. Here are some

things that you men can do while she is growing another human inside of her body. Let me break it down so that you can shine during the gestation and delivery of your child. After that, you're on your own.

First Trimester (Weeks 4-14):

1. Let her sleep, and feed her whatever sounds good as long as it isn't too unhealthy.

2. In early or mid-pregnancy, your "sexual thunder" is not gonna hurt that baby. Mom may be a little more sensitive though. This pearl, by the way, was a quote from one of my favorite dads in my practice. He gave me permission to share.

3. More vaginal discharge is normal, usually. If it doesn't itch or have a foul odor, I wouldn't worry. Recommend that she ask her doctor about it if she's concerned.

4. Google and specifically chat rooms and mom groups are not good for her. She may think they will prevent her from having some untoward fate. They won't prevent complications, but they will encourage paranoia about experiencing every red-herring that could possibly happen. Those chat discussions often disproportionately discuss the negative stories. People with normal pregnancies generally don't post, but they have a substantially greater piece of the pie. Mmm, pie. Don't stress. Remind yourself everything will be fine as often as you remind her that everything will be fine.

5. Regarding her breasts: Look, don't touch, or touch carefully. Her mountains or (as in my case) hills, will be cute, but also a little to very sensitive. Oh, and her breasts will likely deflate later and her nipples will change, but that is life. Your baby is worth it.

Second Trimester (Weeks 12-ish-28):

6. Recommend that she keep a list of questions for the doctor, or keep it for her. Pregnant ladies forget. Don't say that though. She may not appreciate hearing you say that she is getting more forgetful, but pregnancy brain is real.

7. Rub anything she asks you to, or pay someone else to. Get your minds out of the gutter. I'm talking about a massage. Heads up though, a lot of prenatal massage places want a doctor's note for safety clearance before they will do the massage. A little mother-baby safety mixed with CYA, I'm sure. Another one of my favorite dads

surprised his wife with a massage and got a note from me on the sly a couple of prenatal visits prior.

8. Be present at as many appointments as you can—get your questions answered. Be present for scheduled or impromptu ultrasounds. If schedules prohibit this, ask her to record the heartbeat for you. It is a wonderful sound and a gesture that you care.

9. She may be a little mean sometimes. Give her a little pass. Be like a freshly waxed car, and let some of her momentary lapses in basic human respect roll off of you like water. If she isn't letting up, try peaceful communication tactics. Example: I am trying to help by doing X, is that helping? How can I help more? (Give her the book back for this next couple of sentences.) Ladies, try to be nice. He really is trying and is only concerned about you and the baby's well-being. If he suggests healthy snacks, say thank you. Don't smack them out of his hand. Okay, give him back the book. We're wrapping up soon.

10. If she hasn't thought of it, offer to book her a maternity photo shoot. Be ready to be in the pics. If she already booked one, go willingly. The late-second trimester is a good time for this because she is not yet so big that she gets uncomfortable and grumpy.

Third Trimester (Weeks 28-40 or delivery):

11. Don't be afraid to take classes with her, especially if this is your first baby. CPR and what-to-expect type classes are usually pretty helpful. They are available for a small fee at my hospital. Can't swipe that insurance card for those.

12. Offer to go for a walk or to the gym with her. Remind her that it will help her get through the end of the pregnancy and delivery and be strong and conditioned. This will make her delivery easier. Offer to buy her a pregnancy support belt if she complains of pain in her back or pelvic pressure. If she complains a lot about pain and pressure, make sure she speaks with her doctor about it.

13. You are on car seat duty! You guys should buy it together—she will likely have strong opinions about which one you should have. It is very important that it is installed properly and checked. You would be surprised how easy it is to improperly install a car seat. It happened to me. Find a place that can reliably check your installation. I am told that firehouses Do NOT check them anymore. My hospital has patient attendants who are certified, but

check with your hospital before you assume that the same is true.

14. Back to sex, but now in reference to the term (no longer early) pregnancy. Sex is okay and can help encourage labor at the end of pregnancy. The exact mechanism is very technical, involving prostaglandins and cervical stimulation, but in the moment, none of that matters. Make her feel sexy and appreciated. Do not give her anything or let her give herself anything that will induce or start labor without talking to her doctor. Women get desperate at the end sometimes. Just because it is natural, doesn't make it safe. Protect her and your baby by keeping her from being her own worst enemy.

15. Try to do something for her that you don't normally do—clean something that you wouldn't normally tackle. Organize something that she has been meaning to get to—hang up her clothes that she has been meaning to put on hangers. Buy something that she has been saying that she needs—a new shoe rack, perhaps. Am I the only one who has things I've "been meaning to do?"

D-Day—Early labor and hospital labor:

16. She won't look up with a glimmer in her eyes and say, "It's Time," like in the movies. Labor starts slowly and contractions often take hours to days to get to 5 minutes apart. Feed her and hydrate her before it is time to go to the hospital and have her doctor's number programmed into your phone to check in when you've reached that 5-minute mark or have any concerns.

17. Tell her that she is amazing and you love her. Only say that last part if it's true. This is not a time for false or pretend feelings just because you want to be involved with the baby. That's just my opinion.

18. A "Push Present" is a thing. No matter how she delivers this baby, she carried it for almost a year and she felt every moment. Half of these little crumb snatchers don't even look like their moms. Get her a charm, a massage, a clean house (it's okay to hire someone), or any small token of love to let her know you appreciate what she allowed to happen to her body and mind for your collaborated human. As an adjunct, and this one may seem obvious: Do NOT complain about how long labor or pushing is taking. I had a husband once flop down in a chair next to his pushing wife and fix his mouth to say the words: "Uhh, I am so tired of pushing." He's lucky that his child didn't lose her father in that moment. Don't do it. Oh, and do not eat your delicious smelling food in her room or

come back with the breath of onion and garlic when she is unable to eat.

19. Don't let her leave the house without pants or a skirt. I wouldn't be giving this advice if these things hadn't happened under my watch. She showed up... wearing a robe... and that was it. That was ALL. A robe without a belt, might I add. Also, help her with her shoes because she likely can't reach her feet easily.

20. In the delivery room, there may be a lot of healthcare providers in the room, or there may not be. Take as many pictures as she will allow without being annoying. You can delete them later but you can't go back to get them. Rules: no vagina or nipples in the picture, try to avoid flash photos because they are annoying (take advantage of the delivery bright lights), and ask the nurses about recording rules. My hospital doesn't allow the actual delivery to be photographed or recorded. That's okay though because it would break my No Vagina rule anyway.

Postpartum: Back at home and in your own space.

Protect her postpartum: Protect her from your parents, her parents, and anyone who has too much advice. Being helpful is great and their tips are welcome. At the end of the day, though, it's your baby. Schedule family visits to allow for at least 3-hour naps, and put that phone on silent periodically.

Also, since $150,000 baby gifts are not commonplace (#kanye #kim #beyonce) there are a few things that are good to have in the house when your baby comes home.

• Aquaphor and/or coconut oil for diaper changes. Coconut oil has some skin conditioning and antifungal properties that can help prevent diaper rash, and Aquaphor is the best skin protectant ever for extra sensitive skin. We don't use baby powder anymore because of some health concerns, so these are good options.

• Vitamin D Drops. If she is breastfeeding, babies often need a little more vitamin D to keep their nutrition balanced. Even though breastmilk is liquid gold, that D is often a little lacking. Sunbathing isn't a thing in infancy so your pediatrician will likely recommend supplementation. I liked Dr. Carlson's brand because it was just one drop per day, rather than the multiple required by some other brands. #unpaidendorsement

• Lots and lots of baby socks of different sizes from infant to 1 year. My kids ran through socks like diapers. You lose them. You drop them. You don't put away laundry and can't find the matches in the bag of clean clothes. Keep some spares on hand.

• Babyproofing: Socket protectors, cabinet locks, etc. You won't need them right away, but there is no harm in being prepared.

Okay, run the book back to the mother-to-be, if you don't mind. If you are intrigued about what she's reading about here, the next section is about Laparoscopy. Yeah, thought so.

Laparoscopy

Why do surgeons like doing big surgeries through little incisions? I don't know. We like a challenge? No, seriously folks, we like operating through small holes because patients have less pain and recover faster. This is the appeal of laparoscopic surgery. If I can take something out of your body through 2-3 incisions that are all 1-2 cm long, you will feel better than if I cut a larger 10cm incision. Laparoscopy is used for tubal ligations, evaluating and attempting to treat endometriosis, removing ovarian cysts or whole ovaries, removing fibroids in certain circumstances, or removing the uterus in some circumstances.

This surgery is always done in an operating room (unlike some procedures and surgeries that can be done in our office) and requires general anesthesia. That is the type of anesthesia that paralyzes your muscles and requires a breathing tube to breathe for you. Don't worry, though. Anesthesiologists train for years to keep you alive during these procedures. You are in good hands. You need to be paralyzed because the procedure process requires filling the abdomen with air. That gas-filled bloated belly requires the muscles to be completely flabby Abby relaxed (no offense, Abby.)

Any procedure has risks, so experience can definitely matter. If you are so bold, ask your doctor about their history with the procedure, if they say they have had complications, listen to what they did to get out of those sticky situations. I am not saying reward your doctor for having had complications, but listen to see if their complications indicate they've done a lot of procedures in the past. I appreciate it when a doctor knows how to get everyone out of situations safely.

Lesion

Are you looking for more about lumps and bumps in

personal places? Did you start in the Bump section and get sent here? I'm sorry; it's not a wild goose chase. I just ended up writing my comprehensive explanation of all things lumping, bumpy and private in the Things section. This is the last time that I'll send you to another aisle or transfer your call. I promise.

Life and Love

Not the infamous LIKE culture. I am talking about LIFE and LOVE. I make the distinction because hooking up commonly involves some sort of LIKE. That LIKE life can lead to a Pandora's Box of emotions. I won't spend too much time on this particular subject in THIS book. I have a whole book in the works about emotional preservation. It centers around valuing your own LIFE and LOVING yourself enough to not let LIKE define you.

Why do I feel the need to tackle this subject as a gynecologist? Well, I see and care for women from all walks of life. I have observed many states of mind and what sometimes appear to be demonstrations of self-worth. A recurrent theme goes a little something like this, "He LIKED me enough to swipe right, but not enough to get to know me." Over time, this can be destructive to a woman's emotional well-being and affect how she treats future relationships.

I know we haven't made it to the P's yet, but the Powerful Nia series, though written for children, is my love letter to the women of the next generation to love themselves above anyone else, except God. We all experience let downs and challenges, but I want my daughter and her generation to be their own biggest fans. I once wrote a social media post for the 4th of July asking everyone to "Be Your Own Fireworks." That way, no one can define you and make you feel like less of yourself.

Long ago, in the first The Best Man movie, Murch told a young stripper, played by the fabulous Regina Hall, "If I didn't define myself for myself, I would be crunched into other people's fantasies for me and eaten alive," a quote by Audre Lorde. The Best Man was a defining movie for me. We played Cameo's "Candy" at MY wedding because of that movie.

Lubrication

Reminder: At the time that I am writing this chapter I have

not received promise of payment or actual payment for recommending or promoting any products. That means, if I recommend something, it's solely because I have evidence or experience in my practice that it works. Sometimes I have personal experience, but sometimes I use feedback from countless patients as well.

For sex, water-based K-Y jelly and Astroglide are my most popular. I don't have a preference, but people with the tendency to be sensitive down in that region need to stay away from the fragranced, hot and cold, promises-to-have-the-orgasm-for-you lube. Stick with a basic water-based selection.

For vaginal dryness: Vaginal dryness that results from menopause is sometimes hard to treat. Some women don't want to take hormone pills or rub hormones on private or not-private places. A hormone-free vaginal moisturizer that I recommend frequently is called Replens. It is a long-acting moisturizer, so it is not intended to be used just for intercourse. These are just some options. #yourenotalone

6
DON'T MAKE ME OVER

M.

Makeup

You may take a lot of lessons from me. When it comes to makeup application, this is not a lesson that you will be learning here in this book. You can, however, laugh at my ignorance of the subject. I began learning how to wear lipstick as a 35-year-old adult with a husband and three kids. Here is one of my favorite Facebook makeup posts:

New Lips Round 1. Go go gadget Prime. I feel like a little girl about to play dress up. They criticized the King of Pop for Neverland Ranch, but the man missed his childhood being in one of the biggest singing groups of all times. Well, like him (smh), I missed my 20s being in med school and residency. These formative years of makeup development (still smh) were replaced with books, babies, and b-aginas. Could it

be that all this time I thought people said I looked young because of my black that don't crack when, in fact, it was my virgin Alicia-Keys-makeup-free face, which was not an intentional statement, but rather a sign of being ill-equipped? Well, now if you see me in my birthday face (makeup-free like the day I was born) it will be intentional because I'm slowly learning how to do the daggon thang!

Freshly exfoliated, primed, lined and colored (watch it)...

I still consider myself a makeup novice. Which is fine with me because I have always said that I want people to be more familiar with my baseline face. What's my baseline face? It's not my just-woke-up face, but rather my makeup-free face. That way, when you see me with makeup on, you are pleasantly surprised by how nice I can look. The converse to that is for you to see me all of the time with makeup on, but then on a lazy day or one when I had to rush out of the house to deliver a baby, I show up bare-faced, and you say, "DAYUM, WHAT IN THE HELL HAPPENED TO YOU," in full A Different World Ron Johnson voice. Call me Alicia Keys who can't play the piano...or sing very well...and who isn't Alicia Keys but just doesn't wear makeup very often.

Mastitis

This is a breast infection that is usually linked to breastfeeding. What can happen when a woman is lactating, meaning producing milk, is that occasionally milk ducts become clogged. Within a few hours or days, an infection can set in which is extremely painful and often accompanied by fevers and chills. The preliminary clogged duct can also be painful and cause low-grade temperature rises. If that engorged area is unclogged with heat and frequent emptying, sometimes mastitis can be avoided. The most important hallmark is fever over 100.4 degrees.

Mastitis can also occur in non-pregnant women but it is extremely rare. I recommend imaging with ultrasound or mammogram if you develop mastitis at a time when you are not actively producing milk for a baby.

If you suspect mastitis, check your temperature. If you don't have an actual fever yet, pump every 2 hours, use warm compresses and try to massage the tender area to relieve the blockage. If the situation is beyond remedy, or none of those tactics works, call your doctor and plan to take an antibiotic consistently for 10-14 days. Keep feeding and pumping to keep the milk flowing. If the situation still doesn't improve quickly, you may need imaging to make sure an abscess has not formed.

The take-home message: Mastitis sucks.

Masturbation

You'll go blind.

Just kidding. You won't go blind unless you pull an HBO Insecure Season 2 Issa/Daniel number, and a sharpshooter hits you with a spermy egg white full of Chlamydia, and you leave it there. I'm not even sure that would lead to permanent damage, but let's not take any chances. Flush with water, Issa, and watch for redness, irritation and discharge. That wasn't even a masturbation scene, but it was entertaining.

My only masturbation advice is two-fold. If you have never had a clitoral orgasm, you may want to check out the scene down there and see if you can produce your own climax. Then you'll have a better positive feedback system for a partner to help get your jollies. If YOU don't even know what leads to your internal explosion, how can you expect for a partner to be proficient? You may have to lead this parade. It would help if you know where it's going. (That was a lot of euphemisms* in a row, but my mom may be reading this, so I'm sorry.)

*A euphemism is a mild or indirect word or expression substituted for one considered to be too harsh or blunt when referring to something unpleasant or embarrassing.

The second-fold (my advice was two-fold, remember?) is that, like anything that makes you feel good, masturbation can be addicting. Surprised? I mean if people can be addicted to food or porn, of course, masturbation could make the list. Know your limitations. Obsession can possibly lead to harm if things become too aggressive or if toys (if you go there) are not cleaned well or stored properly. I don't want to belabor this point, but I'm just saying that too much of a good thing is a "thing."

No, no, I can't leave it at that. This sounds like I'm anti-masturbation. I'm not, and there are some suspected health benefits that can be derived, including relaxation, cardiovascular health, and for men, even up to a 30% decrease in prostate cancer. And it feels good. Do your thing ladies, just in moderation. More on the orgasm discussion in the big O Section. #punlife

Men

There's a lot for you guys in the L's. Go back to Labor and Delivery and enjoy a whole section targeted toward helping a significant other through pregnancy and delivery from the man's perspective.

One piece of advice: If you are concerned about your wife's or significant other's vagina, remind her to see her gynecologist and dentist for routine preventative screening. I mention the dentist because I believe that if you mention the two together, she may just think that you value preventative health maintenance instead of targeting her lady problem. Your Google research about how to freshen up her vagina will NOT be well received in 9 out of 10 women. This little kernel of advice comes from the Uber driver who asked my Gyneco-(b)Logic partner in crime, Dr. Shelly Agarwal, what he could tell his wife to make her vagina fresher. Pick your battles and choose your words carefully, sir.

Let's talk "pull-out" for a second. It is a topic that comes up more frequently with my male friends than with my female friends or patients. I think that it is because a man loves the feeling of an un-condom-ized bone. Yes, I said bone. I'm trying to invoke my inner "dude" to talk to the guys. Is it working? Anyway, if a man thinks that he can have sex and not get his partner pregnant WITHOUT needing to wear a condom, he may be intrigued. Here is the problem: The pull-out method is a numbers game. Assuming that every time, the pull-out was perfectly timed and consistent, only 4 in 100 women will get pregnant within a year. That is what is known as perfect use. Then there is typical use: the stats reflecting human error that happens from time to time. With typical use, 22 in 100 women will get pregnant in 1 year. This number continues to grow with every year that this method is used.

Think back to the days when your parents made you watch Wheel of Fortune on the family TV. Am I dating myself? There were about 100 triangular panels on that wheel. Imagine that wheel, instead of having money on it, has pregnancy interspersed on random panels. With typical use, pull out would put pregnancy on 1 in 5 panels. If you were hoping for a jackpot on the roulette wheel, you would play with 1 in 5 odds. You would play a lot because hitting a win with 1 in 5 odds is very doable. That's if you want to hit (couldn't help it). Is that the kind of birth control that you want, though? Whether spinning for $5000 or not, do not underestimate pregnancy or STD stats on that wheel. Choose a birth control method that either takes pregnancy off the wheel (abstinence is the only one there) or leaves, like, 1 out of 100 chances, unless you want that jackpot.

Menstrual Cycle

A period, a cycle, aunt Flo, on the rag, the ketchup packet, and every other reference to suggest bleeding as it relates to that "time of the month." I got the "ketchup packet" from a patient. I literally laughed out loud.

All vaginal bleeding is not a menstrual cycle. For example, if a woman is on certain types of birth control, bleeding is just "comfort blood". Comfort blood is a term I coined to reference cyclic bleeding that is caused by birth control and gives a woman reassurance that she isn't pregnant. It isn't present for any other purpose. If a woman is not on birth control, every month is a potential pregnancy. She ovulates, that egg is released from the ovary and travels down the fallopian tube toward the uterus. If it isn't fertilized, it travels out of the body unnoticed, and the bed that had been made for it, her uterine lining, is shed in a bloody babbling brook, stream, or waterfall for some. In that setting, the period signals to the person that she is not pregnant.

If hormonal birth control is in play, depending on the type, a woman may not ovulate and won't NEED to have a period every month. Some want it though (#notme), I could write a whole chapter or a whole book about this. Instead of spending time being boring, let's just tackle two common questions: When is it okay to have a period? And when is it okay not to?

It is okay to have a period every 21-35 days when off of birth control. Anything more often or less frequent than that is worth discussing with your doctor to check for possible hormonal or structural causes. The most common cause for a missed period is pregnancy, so feel free to run that test at home first. If you are off of birth control and have periods and don't want to get pregnant but want to have sex, the best idea is to initiate some sort of RELIABLE birth control (meaning get out of here with your rhythm, pull-out, sometimes-condoms foolishness). Otherwise, get on prenatal vitamins and start a baby registry. Go check out the Contraception section for more about your options.

When is it okay to NOT have a period? When you are on hormonal birth control. Whether you take the pill, the shot, a hormonal IUD, the ring or anything with hormones in it, you can skip your period and not be unsafe or unhealthy. I delve more into the reasons why in the PCOS and the Questions sections. So as to not be redundant, check that out for more about the different reasons a person would not have a period.

Menopause is also a time when it is okay to not have a period. In fact, if you have stopped having periods, but then they start again, that is a problem. I feel a Segue coming on...

Menopause

Mini is a lady who we all know. Her full name is Min E. Pause. Ms. Pause may be your friend, your neighbor, or she may even be you. We will tackle some of her medical issues in the section entitled, Old. #YesIWentThere

First, let us define menopause. Menopause is defined as twelve consecutive months of being vaginal blood-free. This coupled with intermittent hot flashes, night sweats, sometimes weight changes, and being 45-years-old or older are good signs of this diagnosis. For clarity, menopause can actually occur in anyone 40 years or older. If it occurs before the age of 40, it is considered premature ovarian failure. In addition, there are other hormonal disorders, for example, those caused by thyroid malfunction, that can mimic menopausal changes. Some women will actually bleed more in perimenopause, which is the time when the hormonal fluctuations have started but you haven't made it the full period-free 12 months to reach menopausal nirvana (is that a thing?). There are 3 things that every woman entering the "change" should know:

1. Bleeding irregularities, especially bleeding between periods and heavy bleeding, should be evaluated by a gynecologist. I don't mind if your periods space out, but too frequent bleeding or high volume bleeding warrant a check-up. #NoSurpiseThere

2. Once a woman is confirmed to be menopausal, bleeding should NOT start back up again. In other words, if you have not bled for 12 months, then start bleeding again, that isn't a period. That is abnormal bleeding. #AgainCallYourDoctor

3. The vagina will go through trials and tribulations, but with some special considerations, you can keep it as happy and healthy as possible. Supplemental hormones and other medication can help with vaginal dryness and pain with intercourse. Laser therapy can also help to restore the natural vaginal tissue and lubrication. Talk to your doctor about those options. #surprisesurprise

I'll talk more about bone health in the Osteoporosis section. Walking a lot and having a diet that is robust in calcium are good places to start. Mini can be a jerk sometimes, but most of the time, she is manageable—sometimes, with a little help.

Michigan

Go Blue! (That's for my husband, Dr. Ed McDonald, and friends.)

Mosquito

Who is Zika? Well, it's not that girl who lived down the block; it's a virus. This virus is transmitted by mosquito bites and causes mild, cold-like symptoms in those exposed, but in select populations, the implications are large. Here are a few facts you should know and can share with family and friends to try to keep loved ones safe.

Pregnant women and women attempting to become pregnant beware. The biggest concern for those exposed to the Zika virus is the possibility of causing severe birth defects in unborn children. Women infected with the Zika virus during pregnancy can deliver infants with microcephaly and brain abnormalities. Microcephaly is an abnormally small head and brain under-development. While it is possible for children with this condition to be of normal intelligence, developmental delays often affecting things such as speech, movement and balance are more common. Those at greatest risk of having a baby with microcephaly and malformations appear to be women who were infected with Zika during the first trimester of their pregnancy.

How do you get it? Mosquito bites. Because there is no vaccine or prevention other than mosquito bite prevention, nor is there any treatment for this virus, the Center for Disease Control (CDC) and American College of Obstetrics and Gynecology (ACOG) recommend postponing travel to affected areas if you are pregnant or planning to be within the next 3 months. (These are the recommendations as of 2019.) The geographical locations of concern are on the CDC website. Check there for updates before booking travel plans.

Only 1 in 5 people infected with the Zika virus become

symptomatic. The symptoms are fever, rash, joint pain and red irritated eyes, similar to pink eye. Symptoms usually only last several days to one week and are typically mild. Severe symptoms requiring hospitalization are rare. The CDC recommends blood testing for pregnant women with symptoms during or shortly after traveling to an affected area.

What if you have no symptoms but recently traveled to an affected area? Pregnant women who have returned from affected countries should tell their healthcare providers so that testing and closer surveillance of the fetus can be initiated. This often includes serial ultrasound to look for signs of brain malformation. It is believed that men can hold the Zika virus in their semen for up to three months, so protected intercourse or abstinence is important during that time period if you are pregnant or could become pregnant. Visitors to countries affected by the virus should wear long sleeves and long pants, and use insect repellent containing DEET.

The Zika virus can have severe lifelong implications for unborn children. Cancel booked travel to these affected areas if you are pregnant and diligently prevent pregnancy if travel is unavoidable. Let's hope you bought the travel insurance, but even if you didn't, your unborn baby's life is worth a lot more than the money lost.

For more information about Zika and other infectious diseases, please check the Center for Disease Control website, CDC.gov, regularly.

Motherhood

Supermom, I am not. I do the best that I can to keep them alive on a daily basis. I told my husband a few months ago that my third adult book was going to be entitled Confessions of a Failing Mother. He didn't like that title because he disagreed with the idea that I am failing. He is so supportive. But I came up with the title as I was standing over my 1-year-old's fresh stool in the middle of my living room floor while my 8- and 5-year-olds looked at us, shaking their heads. I think my 5-year-old even threw out a "How did you let that happen, mom?" Thanks, son. #failing

I was fortunate to have been interviewed about motherhood, which for a few moments let me think that I had this all together. I am including the interview here to give you some parenting tricks and reassure you that we all go through similar challenges. It also is a reminder to me that I do all right in this parenting thing from time to time:

Interviewer: How do you find that mom who can help you rock the parenting thing? Should you join new mom groups? Talk about meeting people soon after having a baby.

Me: People, moms included, can completely demolish a woman's confidence as a new parent. By the way, I am a mother of three. To find that mom who can be a mentor, I looked for parents who have kids who listen to them. If I see a mom whose son or daughter speaks to them consistently in a disrespectful tone or doesn't listen to appropriately delivered requests (not yelling, but speaking firmly and not wavering), that is not the mom that I need to spend a lot of time with. Similarly, that child may not be one that my kid needs to spend a lot of time with. Even when they are small, you can tell a toddler whose parent has absolutely no expectations for obedience versus the child who is just rambunctious, and the parent is just doing the best they can. I'd rather hang with the latter.

Mom's groups can be extremely supportive, but when the culture is one of comparing birth stories, breast milk quantities and the latest milestones in a "your child isn't doing that yet?" tone, that can be unhealthy for a new mom. I'll take a group that dishes about how hard parenting can be and supports each other's struggles over the whose-kid-is-best group any day. Also, I prefer hanging with moms who know that they cannot do it all. Dads can help too, AND they aren't always wrong in their style of help. I have learned a lot from mothers who allow husbands/fathers to do tasks their own way and realize, *gasp*, that the tasks can still get done.

Interviewer: What qualities do you want to find in your mom mentor?

Me: I want my mom mentor to be someone with a lifestyle similar to mine. Every once in a while I'd like to have a girls' night with a working mom who still finds the time to love her husband and take care of herself. It's much easier than finding time to have coffee with a mom who doesn't work and who marvels in a slightly judgmental fashion about "how you do it all without worrying about your kids all of the time." My ability to make it to a few field trips per year is a miracle. If another mom can pick up her kids every day with no use for aftercare AND make it to all of the field trips, more power to her, but she can't be in my closest inner-circle. Mom-guilt is a real thing. The kids find perfect ways to dish it out liberally, often to get more toys or junk. I don't need it to come, even subliminally, from another mom.

Interviewer. Why is having a mom mentor so important?
Me: Everything in life is relative. I hate spending the night away from my kids. What if they wake up? What if they need me in the still, quiet night? When I have to spend the night away from them because of a hospital shift, I remind myself that there are mothers in the armed services who have to leave their families for months on end. I am reminded that if those women can survive those tours away from family, I can survive a 12-hour shift. It is that perspective that works to keep me going.

When I see a mom at school, and I can tell that she is doing the best she can (hair isn't perfect, clothes aren't super trendy), I feel better about my tossed up hair and not-trendy outfit that was all I could muster up to get all of us out of the house this morning. I once wrote a post on a Facebook doctor mom's group that said, "It must be nice to be my husband because... I just fed and got all three kids in bed and cleaned the kitchen. He has been finishing his office notes all evening. Now I need to start mine." Instantly, 30 other moms chimed in with their "It must be nice to be my husband" contributions. I felt validated and not alone. We all love our spouses, but we share in the occasional unequal burden of being working moms in high-demand jobs, and it helps.

We can share in things that each of us can use for our kid's enrichment. One playdate with some friends resulted in us signing our boys up for Kumon, an amazing extracurricular math and reading enrichment program. We had been talking about it for years but talking to parents whose kids were actually doing it and loving it helped push us over the edge. We will hopefully help our kids blossom academically. This is the kind of group I want to hang with. Support, not keeping-up-with-the-Joneses comparison, is what I am looking for.

When I get home today, I need to figure out how to get melted plastic off of the bottom of the oven and off of the oven rack. A refrigerator magnet found its way to the bottom of my metal pizza sheet, and the oven demolished it. Here we go...
#motherhood #stillfailing

My Motto

My motto is: No surprises. Hey, I'm a gynecologist. The last thing that a woman wants during her Gyne exam is to be in the middle of a sentence about her kids' latest accomplishment or her upcoming vacation and get a speculum surprise. Hello! (Like in the old movies). I love to catch up and hear the latest and greatest in my ladies' lives. I consider most of my patients friends—not close, come to my house friends, but more like Facebook acquaintances who I will speak to if I see them in Mariano's. I am pretty chatty, but we can still seamlessly carry out their exam. Mid-sentence, I will interject—"I'm about to do your breast exam," or, pre-Pap, I'll throw out a "You're about to feel me touch and feel lots of pressure. If anything hurts, you let me know. You should not feel pain, but pressure is normal. Now, where are you all going on vacation?"

Pressure and pain are sensations that are often confused in the genital region. I always try to set the expectation that the pelvic exam is not comfortable, but it shouldn't hurt. Sometimes women are afraid that the exam is going to hurt, even if it doesn't. Fear and shock can go hand in hand. Scary movies couple surprise with fear. If I can take the surprise factor out of the exam and set reasonable expectations, then my patient has a reasonable chance of not hating her gynecologist forever. #nosurprises

Myomectomy

Fibroids are, in most cases, benign growths on the uterus. Especially in the African American community, the risk of a woman developing fibroids in her lifetime is 80%. The lifetime risk in Caucasian women is 70%. I found out that I had fibroids in college. My gynecologist thought he felt something during the exam and sent me for an ultrasound, which confirmed the presence of a baseball in my uterus. That was cool, though. It didn't bother me. Fast forward to my pregnancy with my first son in 2008. Maybe it was the same original fibroid, or maybe a different one, but it grew to about 10 centimeters, about the size of a grapefruit and you could feel it when you touched (with permission) my belly. My co-residents called it my second baby head.

After my pregnancy was over, one of my docs was like, "Okay, Wendy, when can you take some time off so that we can get this out?" I was like, "Um…let me check my scheeeduuuullleeee and get baaaccckkk toooo youuuuu." That statement was very slow and high pitched, which in Wendy-speak means, I'm not going to check my schedule and not going to get back to you because you need to keep your knife off of my uterus. Hold up. This is not a statement of my being anti-surgery or anti-myomectomy, but more so me being anti-unnecessary surgery or unindicated myomectomy. My bleeding wasn't heavy, I didn't have any appreciable pressure on my bowels or bladder, I didn't look pregnant (no more than any other woman who has had a baby), so there was no need for me to go under the knife at that time. If any of those symptoms had developed, well, THEN we could have a conversation about a myomectomy, or fibroid removal, and the specific route to carry this out.

There are three types of myomectomy: abdominal, laparoscopic and hysteroscopic myomectomy. Abdominal means removal through a laparotomy, which is a horizontal or vertical cut on the skin, and removal in the way that a baby is removed during a C-section. This is most commonly performed on women with several large and bulky fibroids that are too large for removal through the vagina alone, and also for women with previous abdominal surgeries and scar tissue that would increase the risk of complications with a laparoscopic surgery. A laparoscopic myomectomy removes fibroids using the small laparoscopic skin incisions. This requires extensive experience and patience. Performing a laparoscopic myomectomy is like trying to peel an orange, and not an easy-to-peel Cutie, in a fishbowl using long tweezers AND looking at a TV screen at the image from a camera in the fishbowl AND trying to stop the orange from losing as little juice as possible. See what I am saying?

The last type of myomectomy is a hysteroscopic myomectomy. This is good for smaller fibroids that are in the cavity of the uterus. But wait, Dr. Wendy, you just said that you don't remove small fibroids. No, I said that I don't remove fibroids that aren't causing trouble. Fibroids in the cavity of the uterus are often discovered because the woman is having heavy or irregular bleeding. They can also be found during an investigation for infertility. These fibroids can be shaved down and removed by putting a woman to sleep and inserting a camera into the uterus through the vagina and cervix. (See Hysteroscopy.)

Surgery is not the only way to treat fibroids. One can also

have a uterine artery embolization, which is a procedure performed by a radiologist to occlude the arteries that give blood supply to the uterus. This procedure is often able to slow or stop heavy bleeding and shrink the size of the fibroids by about 30%. Other options include symptom management with medication to slow bleeding or stabilize the growth of fibroids. Ultrasound treatment, called Focused Ultrasound Surgery (or FUS), is also an option in a few medical centers in the US.

Take-home message: I am more than happy to help you to control or remove your fibroids if necessary. My fibroid motto, however, remains: If they don't bother you, they don't bother me.

N.

Nipples

Did you ever notice that the nipples in cartoons look like spinning circles? I was watching Hercules with my kids, and I was straight up mesmerized by Zeus's hypnotic nipples. His pecs were just so big. Then I was thinking, could you give Zeus a Titty Twister? Like I know he was supposed to be immortal, but even the king of the mythical gods probably had some sensitive nipples.

Nipples are important for breastfeeding. This is where the baby extracts "liquid gold", known as colostrum and breastmilk. I wrote my tips for breastfeeding back in the Breastfeeding section, but let's just talk nipple care for a minute.

The Inverted Nipple—If they have never been inverted, meaning the nipples start to dive inward rather than protrude outward, this can be a sign of breast disease such as cancer. If you have always had craters rather than mounds, then don't worry, you are unique in every way. If you ever do decide that you want to feed a baby sweet, off-white nectar from the fruit of your bosom, you can sometimes use a manual or electric breast pump to evert the nipple. Nipple shields can also be used to give a baby something to hold on to when trying to nurse.

Latch is not just a dope Sam Smith song. It is the grip that a baby has during feeding. If that grip isn't correct (Oh, the pain!), a poor latch in breastfeeding can feel like a nipple stabbed you in the chest, and nipples aren't sharp. IT HURTS. Even a good latch WILL hurt some. Late night feedings where I didn't even want to turn the light on were deemed successful when I felt that characteristic nipple pinch. The point is, some pain is expected with breastfeeding, especially at the beginning. Only if the nipples are significantly cracked or inflamed are medicated or prescription ointments necessary.

What if you are noticing breast discharge/drainage, and you aren't pregnant? The first question to ask is: Is it spontaneous or provoked? What I mean is, do you see it in your bra or do you have to squeeze the nipple to see it? If you always have to squeeze to see it, stop squeezing. The breasts have a feedback system that will make them produce more if stimulated. Leave them alone. If you look into the bra, or no bra depending on how you are rolling, and you see it spontaneously, you may need to wear less irritating bras or shirts. If there is no irritation, but still there is spontaneous discharge, depending on the color and severity it could be nothing, or it could be a sign of a more serious problem, possibly even cancer. See your doctor for any unexplained nipple discharge, especially if it persists after the stimulation stops.

O.

Obstetrician

See Gynecologist. Just kidding.

An obstetrician is a medical doctor who specializes in delivering babies and caring for women in all stages of pregnancy and the postpartum period, which is the six weeks after the baby is born. A midwife can also care for a woman during her pregnancy and deliver her baby. The difference between an obstetrician and a nurse midwife is that midwives can, generally speaking, only take care of low-risk pregnancies. Also, they can only deliver babies vaginally without any intervention. If a pregnancy becomes high-risk or if an operative delivery is needed (vacuum, forceps or C-section) the medical doctor needs to step in to care for the patient.

I have the utmost respect for what midwives do. I do want to point out that just because a midwife cannot perform a C-section, doesn't mean that if you choose to be under a midwife's care, then you won't need a C-section. I am not a trigger-happy doctor. I try to avoid C-section just like any good practitioner. If a labor takes that turn, though, I don't need to tap out with someone to take you through the home stretch. A midwife does need to tap out. Every midwife that I know is super caring and attentive, and they are often breastfeeding experts. Health centers can only afford to employ so many doctors. They can often hire significantly more midwives and nurse practitioners, meaning more patients can be seen and cared for without the healthcare establishment going into the red.

A gynecologist is a medical doctor who specializes in taking care of women, from adolescence to elderly. As a gynecologist, I know a whole lot of information about your lady parts. I know how to keep women healthy and what to do when things go awry. I cannot say that I know everything about your heart, your ears, or your kidneys. An internal medicine doctor is a full body, head-to-toe doctor who cares for women and men and knows generally about every organ system. There are specialists in every body system, from the blood to the brain to the everything. Even though gynecology is considered primary care, I don't exercise my full PCP (primary care physician) potential. I work in a large city with multiple specialists and subspecialists. Because of this, I am not the best person to manage your high blood pressure, your diabetes, or your toenail fungus. I have an internist who I see for my own care. If you let your internist do your Pap smear, make sure that you go to see a gynecologist if it is abnormal. If your Pap is painful, it may be because internists often have only one size speculum. What is a speculum? To S, with you!

A pediatrician is someone who specializes in caring for children from their first newborn arrival through adolescence or teenage years. Now hold on before you start judging my breakdown of what might be common knowledge to some of you. Common isn't always common. That is the point of the book, and you are reading it, too. Un-pause.

A neonatologist is someone who specializes in caring for babies born prematurely or with severe medical issues. They spend a lot of time in the neonatal intensive care unit, also known as the NICU.

A perinatologist, more contemporarily known as a Maternal-Fetal Medicine (MFM) specialist, is a doctor who specializes in caring for high-risk pregnancies. I have to throw in a disclaimer. In my practice working at Prentice Women's Hospital, we have a very close relationship with the MFMs. They disseminate guidelines consistent with ACOG (American College of Obstetricians and Gynecologists) guidelines and common regional practices to keep each doc at our institution practicing within the standard of care. That means though, that many women who are pregnant and diabetic, hypertensive (have high blood pressure), or with any other mild ailment of pregnancy can often be managed by a general OB/GYN. It is only when a patient's medical problems start to get super complicated and "creative" that I become more than willing to transfer care to MFM for further management. We want to keep mom and baby safe as much as mom and baby want to be safe. Obviously, it is every woman's right to choose who will care for her in pregnancy (insurance and politics aside), but I love caring for women during their pregnancies, even those who are high-risk.

Advanced practice nurses include nurses who have at least a Master's degree. Under this category are nurse practitioners, nurse midwives, nurse anesthetists, and clinical nurse specialists. Nurses are amazing in their ability to help keep patients safe and be the eyes and ears for the patient and doctor. I love my nurses. I trust my nurses. Without them, healthcare would be practically impossible.

A doula is not a healthcare provider by profession, but doulas do specialize in helping women navigate the stages of labor and delivery, postpartum, and breastfeeding, in a one-on-one personal way. They help ladies with breathing, concentration and navigating the fear of the unknown. They are known to be helpful to women who want to get through labor without an epidural or medical pain management. That is what Lamaze is/was for. It was to help women control their breathing and survive the intense pains of labor. A doula is like a personal Lamaze coach. For those of us who have no shame about requesting pain management, they may not be quite as helpful. You do have to pay them out-of-pocket. They usually come to your house and help you through the early stages of labor too.

A word of doula caution: you should not use them as, or expect them to be, your anti-C-section. If your baby needs to come out any other way than through your vagina, your doula has no control over that and cannot prevent it. Women with doulas have the same C-section rate as those without. Things that affect your need for a C-section are your baby's health and well-being, your body's ability to get your cervix to 10 centimeters, your pelvis size, your ability to push, and more. Your doula can support you through the process of having a baby, but he or she cannot crawl into your vagina and pull your baby out of your uterus. Too graphic? The point needed to be made.

Old

A patient once told me, "Aging is a choice." I am an '80s baby. 1981, to be exact. I am proud of my age. Every day that I live is a day that I'm not dead, yet. I am not afraid of dying because I trust that my Lord has saved my soul. What I do fear is leaving the land of the living before my children can fend for themselves. If I were childless, take me whenever you're ready, Lord. I know that life and death are out of my control, but if I had my choice, my kids wouldn't have to miss me until their childhood is complete. The thought of this makes me tear up right now. Be grown enough to not have to rely on me for school lunches, afterschool pick-ups, or college student loans. At the rate that college tuition is rising, I won't be able to die until they are retiring. That's cool though. Having three young kids makes me look forward to being a grandmother, so the little ones can go HOME with their OWN parents.

"End of life" is a term used by healthcare professionals to refer to preparations that should be made before that bucket is kicked all of the way over. I'm not talking death panels here. I don't even know what that is. I'm talking about decisions that are put into writing about how you want your life and your stuff to be handled when you can't speak anymore. Sidebar: If I'm alive only because electricity is flowing through a breathing machine, and medications are keeping my heart beating, turn that stuff off. Now, if I fall in a frozen pond and you may be able to bring me back, try. But if my insides are being replaced by monstrous, ruthless cancer cells, let me go.

You best believe (that is colloquial for "you better believe" in case you are unfamiliar) that I will do everything in my power to give my children and those coming after them a head start in life. For those who don't know what I am talking about, there are people who start adulthood with hundreds of thousands of dollars at their disposal, not to be disposed of, but to use for home down payments, educational expenses, etc. I am blessed to have the education and family that I have, but I had to climb down into the ditch of debt to get here. I am still trying to climb my way out. With all of the money and time that I put into rising out of this ditch, if I started on level ground, I'd be taking over the world by now. I am not Pinky or the Brain, but my kids will have the ability to be. When I die, my KIDs are about to get PAID.

"How?" you may ask. Life insurance, investments, etc. I know there are a million ways to invest for the future and for your children. I am still learning the ropes there—aspiring to Double Dutch (Double Dutch is the advanced form of jump rope, get it? Learning the "ropes"). Talk to me in five years when I write a book with my friend Dr. Bonnie Mason all about how to build wealth and financial freedom in an age where many are undereducated about money matters.

In regards to women's health (I probably should have started there), keep in mind that anything you do in young adulthood will have repercussions over time. Your health doesn't get better as you age. If you are steadily gaining weight every year, count on being at higher risk of developing high blood pressure, diabetes, back pain, joint pain, and many other disorders. If you smoke, know that every cancer known to man is more common in people who smoke.

Check this: If you plant a seed in fertile soil, water it at regular intervals, make sure that it has plenty of sunlight and oxygen, it will grow and flourish until its life is done or its season is over. If you plant it, however, in rocks, water it with Kool-Aid, and sit on it all day so that it doesn't see sun or feel oxygen, it may try to grow for a while, but it WILL die, young. I myself am the anti-green thumb, so I don't know why I am using a plant analogy. Like that plant, though, your body requires good decisions MOST of the time to thrive and live for a long time. To those saying, "Well we all die from something…" that is true. I just want to see my kids and grandkids for as long as possible before that sweet chariot carries me home. I don't want to live too long though. If the mainstream rap music these days is any prediction for music of the future, eventually, imma be ready to get up outta here.

Orgasm

I wrote a whole post about this subject in my blog, The Gyneco-(b)Logic. The post was entitled "Sex, Lies and HBO Insecur-ities." It was all about the differences between what efforts result in orgasm from woman to woman. This post was inspired by a curious patient and the Season 2 opener of HBO's Insecure. My patient conversation was with a woman in her late 30's who asked me, as I had my hand on the doorknob on my way out the exam room (a clear marker for the conclusion of our visit), about how she could remedy the fact that she had never had an orgasm. She went on to ask where her G-spot was because her internal medicine doctor told her that I could show it to her. Needless to say, I sat back down.

What Jo-Issa Rae Diop (her government name, and it's pronounced "Jope") has demonstrated in a few sex scenes on Insecure was that Lawrence could easily orgasm without any evidence of Tasha or Issa doing the same. It prompted the following discussion of the stats and science behind the female orgasm. I asked the question, "Are all hookups created equally?" The answer is, no. The following stats are compiled from a number of research studies and data.

Fact #1: Only 25- 50% of women have ever had AN orgasm, let alone multiple orgasms during penetrative intercourse. Said differently, penetrative intercourse alone is unlikely to lead to orgasm in more than half of all women!

Fact #2: Some studies say that up to 10% of women have never had any type of orgasm, vaginal or clitoral. Ever.

Fact #3: Some women can have multiple orgasms from multiple sources, positions, and a cornucopia of styles and efforts. A blessing or a curse? You be the judge.

The Point: If penile-vaginal penetration alone doesn't take you there, you're not broken, or alone.

For more pontification about the G-spot, clitoris and all other things orgasmic, head back to the Anatomy section where all (maybe not all) secrets are revealed. If you have more questions, make an appointment. #ihatetoleaveitlikethat

Osteoporosis

The development of peanut-brittle bones can happen to anyone. It is not just a frail, old, white woman's disease. (No shade to the frail, old women out there. Thanks for reading. Carry on.) The chance of developing osteoporosis is definitely higher in women who are older, Caucasian and of lower body weight (See how I tried to clean that up?), but anyone can develop this disease.

Osteoporosis is a bone disease that causes the bones to become less dense and thus more likely to break. Who remembers the Muppet cartoon, Fraggle Rock? Well, if you don't remember, they were a group of Muppet Baby-like characters that worked in these underground mines. I don't recall what the purpose of their mining was, but who cares, right? To bring this literary distraction back to osteoporosis, imagine that little Muppet miners within our bones were chipping away at the bone over time, just digging little craters and holes throughout this boney matrix. As time progressed, the mine itself would become very fragile and likely start collapsing on itself. That is what osteoporosis does to our bones.

Osteoclasts are like little bone miners who chip away at bone and remove it. What is supposed to happen is that these little cement pourers, called osteoblasts, are supposed to lay down new bone to replace the old removed bone. If the osteoclasts work too well or too quickly, or the osteoblasts underperform, there can be a net deficiency in bone structure which can cause bones to be weak or break. I am talking about breaks in the spine, compression fractures in the feet from something as simple as walking, and definitely hip fractures in the event of a fall.

People who are more likely to develop osteoporosis are elderly women, generally of lower body weights (the 'big girls'/rotund women win this round), women who have diets low in calcium and vitamin D, and women who use steroids long-term, smoke cigarettes or drink excessive amounts of alcohol—three or more "drinks" per day. Osteoporosis aside, three drinks would be considered excessive alcohol in my system. I personally epitomize the term "lightweight". Give me one, and I am truly done.

Prevention ideally should include consuming dietary calcium and vitamin D, as well as performing weight-bearing exercises regularly. Weight-bearing exercise includes anything that bears weight. Talk about defining a word with a word. If you walk, run, lift, press or snatch (for you crossfitters) weights, that puts strain on your bones and tells them to make sure that they are strong. Not bearing weight (sitting, laying around, barely walking, or doing weightless-ish exercise like swimming) doesn't tell your bones to boss up. Bike riding is considered partial weight-bearing. It counts, but not as much as walking, running, elliptical or lifting, unless you are a serious rider like my amazing cousin, Brandon.

I will bet that astronauts would lose bone strength while weightless in outer space. I just took that theory to Google and came back with this little gem: Spaceflight osteopenia refers to the characteristic bone loss that occurs during spaceflight. Astronauts lose an average of more than 1% bone mass per month spent in space.

What can I say? That girl (me) is GOOD! Putting my tooting horn away, a conscious effort to have a healthy diet and to put your body through some healthy physical challenges will reduce the risk of your bones breaking and your life changing. The Mayo Clinic website summarized some consequences of hip fracture in the elderly:

A hip fracture can reduce your future independence and sometimes even shorten your life. About half of people who have a hip fracture aren't able to regain their ability to live independently. Some of the reasons are as follows:

* If a hip fracture keeps you immobile for a long time, the complications can include:
* Blood clots in your legs or lungs
* Bedsores
* Urinary tract infection
* Pneumonia
* Further loss of muscle mass, increasing your risk of falls and injury

Thank you, Mayo Clinic.

The take-home points: Bone loss occurs over time and if not curbed, can lead to pain, loss of height, and most importantly, fractures. Periodic bone mineral density scans once you've reached menopause will let you know where your bones stand (#punlife) and how aggressive you need to be to keep them strong, whether with lifestyle modifications or medication.

Ovaries

I like to call the ovaries the female "balls". Actually, I don't call them that, ever. My sons used to refer to their baby sister's vagina as her "balls" when they accompanied me to change her diaper. They could understand that she didn't have a penis, but surely she still had to have balls.

In classical Latin, ovarius meant "egg-keeper." Wait, WAIT! Don't put the book down. I know that Latin isn't exciting, but it gets better. We have all of the eggs that we'll have for life when we are born. This is different from men's testicles which are constantly making new sperm. Your eggs are as old as you are. More on that in the Infertility section.

The interesting thing about the ovaries is that they can go haywire if they work too long without breaks. True statement: Women who start having periods early, start menopause late, and don't have children have the highest rates of ovarian cancer. Said differently, If you spend years and years cranking out eggs, those gears may just get rusty, and belts can break, and the whole factory can explode. Too dramatic? Conversely, a woman who has children or goes on ovulation inhibiting birth control has a lower risk of developing ovarian cancer. Pregnancy gives the ovaries almost a year to rest and recoup. Hormonal birth control that stops ovulation (so not IUDs, but only the pill, the shot, the ring, the patch, and the arm implant) also reduces ovarian cancer risk. Nobody likes working without breaks. Not even your ovaries!

That sudden, out of nowhere pain that arises two weeks before you expect your period, or just out of nowhere and lasts a few days, could be the pain of ovulation or an ovarian cyst that is twisting or possibly rupturing. I stress the word COULD because there are many other things that can cause sudden abdominal pain. The least likely cause is ovarian cancer, especially for someone who is premenopausal and without a family history of ovarian cancer. Somehow, Google seems to think that ovarian cancer is the most common cause. I think that is Dr. Google's modus operandi (M.O. as we call it). Google likes to present the least likely and yet deadliest possible cause for your search term. Type into the Google search box, press enter, and DIE IMMEDIATELY. I have even been a victim of Google's Internet poison dart. I typed in something so harmless, and Google told me that I had a flesh-eating bacteria. I was like, "For real, Google?"

Ovarian cancer is not an impossibility though, even for the young. It's just not a common possibility. Anyone with abdominal pain that is intense, recurrent or unrelenting, or a change in the size of the abdomen should... you guessed it... see their doctor. Don't forget about the possibilities of constipation and other bowel diseases, bladder issues, kidney stones, and a variety of both physical and psychological possibilities that The Googs (yes, I nicknamed Google) may or may not have mentioned.

The risk of developing ovarian cancer in a woman's lifetime in the general population is 1 in 70. If a woman has a significant family history of ovarian cancer (usually meaning a first- or second-degree relative who had ovarian cancer), she has a higher risk of developing it. Genetic testing may offer some answers regarding risks and screening methods, but even without genetic testing, if you have a family history, your doctor's surveillance should be higher and the threshold for pelvic and breast imaging—ultrasound and/or mammogram—should be lower. Screening ultrasounds aren't very good for diagnosis for women of low risk, but when risk is higher, it makes more sense.

The take-home point about the ovaries is that they are really sneaky and hard to understand sometimes. Imaging can offer some clarity, but they are often very mysterious. I pray for my ovaries every day. I don't actually, but I should. I pray for my health and strength. That includes my ovaries, right?

.

7
PERIODS, PREGNANCY AND MORE POPCORN

P.

Pain: Vulvodynia

Vulvodynia is chronic pain or discomfort around the opening of your vagina (vulva) for which there's no identifiable cause and which lasts at least three months. #MayoClinic definitions are great. Painful intercourse is one of the hardest things to manage as a gynecologist. Young women can have vaginal and vulvar pain with intercourse for many reasons including a tight hymenal ring. A history of abuse can also lead to pain that can be both physical and emotional. After a woman's anatomy is evaluated by a doctor and found to be normal, sometimes physical therapy can reduce pain. If the anatomy is abnormal, the management depends on what is abnormal.

Older women can have vaginal and vulvar pain and dryness because menopause decreases the amount of estrogen in the vaginal area. This leads to something called vulvovaginal atrophy. Vaginal moisturizers (not just lotion, but moisturizers specifically pH balanced for the vagina) can sometimes help with symptoms of dryness. Pain may require physical therapy, hormone therapy and sometimes laser therapy.

Estrogen and estrogen-like hormones can also help women with menopause-related vaginal pain. Those administered topically (through the skin or vagina) and orally (swallowed) have various pros and cons, risks and benefits that should be discussed with a healthcare provider. Cancer risks vary with the type of medication, the dose of the medication, and your personal history and family history.

You may not have to live with vaginal and vulvar pain. See your gynecologist or a pelvic floor specialist for help. Unfortunately, the problem isn't always solved completely or easily, but I consider improvement in symptoms a small victory.

Pap Test

My patients have told me that they don't like when I call them on the phone. It's not that they don't like me, but rather they have learned to expect that normal results will come electronically or from my medical assistant. Abnormal results, however, will come directly from me. "I'm calling to tell you that your Pap came back abnormal." "My what?" "Your Papanicolau test." "My Papanico-what?" Let's break things down from the basics to the details.

1.   The Pap test looks for pre-cancerous cells on the cervix. These cells are graded by level from normal, to slightly abnormal (atypical and low grade), to significantly abnormal (high grade), to cancer. You can rest assured that if your doctor calls saying you have an abnormal Pap, you don't have cancer. Otherwise, he or she would have said, "You have cancer." Pap testing can be done from as frequently as every 6 months, to as infrequently as every 2-3 years or more in some cases. You and your doctor can discuss how often your Pap should be done.

2.   The Pap test is a screening test that randomly collects a sample of cells from the cervix. If abnormal cells are detected, often a more targeted test is indicated to determine if the Pap accurately represents the cells of your cervix. That targeted test is called a colposcopy. The Colposcopy section goes into greater detail about this test.

3.   HPV, or Human Papillomavirus, is the virus that causes precancerous changes on the cervix. It is also the virus that causes genital warts, though different strains are responsible for warts. HPV is tested as an adjunct to certain Pap results and is routinely tested every few years in women over the age of 30.

4.   If you test positive for HPV, you will never know when, where and from whom you contracted it. Men aren't tested for HPV. Imagine that your Pap is like that T-Rex in Jurassic Park, the first movie. It only saw the people if they moved. Similarly, the Pap will only detect HPV if it is "moving", or replicating. HPV could have been present for years even with normal testing, but if it was dormant in a small quantity, it may not have been detected.

5.   HPV does not necessarily stay forever. It is a virus that your body can, in theory, fight off and destroy. Staying healthy and eliminating or minimizing exposure can help your body to have the immune strength to fight this virus. I stated that you cannot know a partner status, but condom use can at least decrease potential exposure.

There is an FDA approved vaccine for HPV. It protects against the 9 most common and aggressive strains of HPV. It is most effective if administered BEFORE exposure, meaning girls and boys should ideally get the vaccine before the onset of sexual activity. Getting the vaccine does not mean you can skip Paps (#sorrynotsorry), and you should still see your Gynecologist at least annually. As of 2018, the vaccine is recommended for women AND MEN from adolescence through the age of 45.

Rarely does someone get cervical cancer if they follow the screening guidelines and recommendations from their doctor. Even if you get that call about an abnormal Pap, if you do your part and follow up for testing as recommended, you can avoid devastating results and stay safe.

Pelvic Floor

This is the muscle and ligament complex that supports the vagina, uterus, bladder, cervix, and rectum. Basically, it keeps things—pelvic organs, urine, gas, stool—from falling out of place, something called prolapse. The pelvic floor can be well supported due to genetics and/or Kegel exercises, or it can relax and become more stretchy, allowing for prolapse.

Kegel exercises strengthen the pelvic floor muscles to help women hold in urine or gas when it tries to escape. These muscles can become a little traumatized (no pun intended) after pregnancy and childbearing. They can also stop working to the best of their ability as we age. I see so many women entering their menopausal years who have more and more issues with bladder control and leakage. It's quite common.

The pelvic floor can also be a location for pain. The cause of persistent pelvic pain is not always clear, which can make treatment challenging. Constipation, bladder pain, nerve and ligament inflammation and many uterine and ovarian issues can cause pain. As a gynecologist, I discuss the patient's symptoms, I do an exam, I sometimes check an ultrasound and sometimes other laboratory tests to begin the evaluation. Can Google do that? Can It? How Sway? Okay, sorry, down from my soapbox, again. On to more details about pelvic pain.

Pelvic Pain

Pelvic pain sucks.

No, I am not going to drop the mic and move on like that. I want to, though. There are few ailments that I don't like to treat. Chronic pelvic pain is one of them. The reason is that most medical problems in my field are relatively fixable. You have a urinary tract infection, a yeast overgrowth, a pregnancy? I can deliver you from those and help you to bounce back. Chronic pelvic pain, on the other hand, is sometimes not as easily managed and treated.

As I mentioned in the previous section, the uterus, ovaries, bowels, bladder, nerves and fascia can all be direct causes of pain. The evolution and characteristics of symptoms, in combination with a physical exam and sometimes ultrasound, can help with the diagnosis. Treatment depends on the suspected cause but can range from birth control to steroid injections to laparoscopy when indicated. Pelvic floor physical therapy can also many times give women some relief—yes, that is a thing. If you have chronic pelvic pain, talk to your doctor about more in-depth options like consultation with a gastroenterologist, PT or laparoscopy, if the standard birth control or pain medications aren't helping.

Penis

Not my parts. Not in this book. If you are interested in circumcision, that section is in the Cs. Moving on…

Period

See Menstrual Cycle, period. #areyoutiredofmeyet?

Placenta

Well, the placenta looks like a big blood sausage. No, for real! Google break: Search blood sausage in Google Images. Now search placenta and tell me that a placenta with the membranes and all of its texture doesn't look like a blood sausage. What? Are you upset that I have ruined your appetite for blood sausage? You don't eat blood sausage, do you? (It's probably delicious, but I have yet to go there myself.)

The placenta is the source of oxygen and nutrition for a growing baby. When an embryo first implants into the wall of the uterus, the placenta forms and connects with the umbilical cord, which then enters the baby at the umbilicus (the infamous belly button). It is unlike any organ. The placenta is a place of transfer of life-sustaining materials, but mom and baby's blood never mix. Imagine that you ordered some food for delivery—let's say it is a Chicago Style deep dish spinach pizza, only because I'm hungry and would love one of those right now. Anyway, the delivery person arrives at your door, but to receive the food, you have to go get your own plate or container. The delivery person has to take the pizza and the salad out of the box (yes, I do try), and you have to put the food in your own containers before you can bring it into your own house. The placenta is like that. Mommy brings the nutrition and oxygen right up to the placenta, then the placenta has to repackage it and give it to the baby.

This means that a lot of things are not directly passed to the baby. For example, the baby doesn't "like" the food you just ate. He or she can't taste the seasoning on your pizza. He or she is feeling the sugar from your ice cream but does not know the flavor. That's your craving. Don't blame the baby for that. Some things can pass to the baby, though. HIV, in some cases Herpes, blood type antibodies (this is why it matters if your blood type is negative, like A negative or O negative) can all cross the placenta's barrier to possibly affect the baby.

Women with medical problems like high blood pressure and diabetes can also have placentas that don't function well. When a placenta doesn't function well, the baby can be at risk. Because of this, delivery is often scheduled for the best time to ensure the safety of baby and mom, even if that means that an induction of labor or C-section is needed at or before the due date. If the placenta doesn't come out of the uterus in its entirety after baby delivery, a woman can lose excessive amounts of blood. This is called retained products of conception. Sometimes medication or surgical removal is necessary.

I can only write about placentas for so long before I need to cut the cord, (#youknowme) but I will touch on placental encapsulation in the Postpartum Depression section. Let's keep cooking... #really?

Polycystic Ovarian Syndrome (PCOS)

PCOS is an evil, conniving disease. Those are strong words for a disease, but I don't use them without meaning them. Any disorder of the ovaries that will make you gain weight, then make the weight gain worsen the disease like some terrible snowball that nobody wants to play with, is just messed up.

Yes, this disorder causes not only insulin resistance, which leads to ease in weight gain and difficulty with weight loss, but it also causes the ovaries to malfunction and not release an egg at regular intervals. This is known as anovulation and it causes a substantial decrease in fertility and can predispose a woman to develop precancerous and cancerous changes in the uterus. It is just wrong on so many levels.

A cure? Not so much. If a woman can lose weight, ovarian function can sometimes improve. When weight gain isn't her vice, the ovaries can be fooled into functioning with medication and lifestyle changes. Keep in mind, functioning ovaries mean that they release eggs, so if you aren't ready to get pregnant, you don't want that. I repeat, if you are NOT trying to get pregnant, please don't try to make your ovaries work just for the sake of "curing PCOS". You have to think of this syndrome like your natural hair color. You can rock it, but sometimes you may want to change it up for an event or to not look so old. #Iseeyou. You aren't going to "cure" it, but you can modify it.

In the meanwhile, when you are NOT trying to get pregnant, you can keep your uterus safe from overgrowth and abnormal uterine lining growth by using hormonal contraceptives— the progesterone-containing IUD, birth control pills, the Depo-Provera shot. Pick your pleasure.

If you don't want to get too technical, stop reading this section right now. This is where I delve deep into when it is okay to have a period and when it is okay not to. It is OKAY to not have a

period when:
- You are on hormonal birth control, OR
- You are pregnant (duh), OR
- You are breastfeeding

It is NOT okay to NOT have a period when:
- You are not pregnant, AND
- You are not breastfeeding, AND
- You are not on hormonal birth control

When not on hormonal birth control, the uterine lining may not be shedding because of a discoordination between the brain and the ovaries. In a normal cycle, the brain signals the ovaries to release an egg, and if that egg isn't fertilized, the egg is expelled, and the uterine lining is shed in menstrual flow, like changing the sheets after customers check out of a hotel room.

If the ovaries are not prompted by the brain to release an egg, the uterus doesn't know when or how to change the sheets. The uterine lining—the sheets in my analogy—gets all murky and dusty and abnormal, and before you know it, you got bed bugs. Okay, I may have taken that one a little too far, but the abnormality of the uterine lining is the point. If it doesn't shed at some point, it has an opportunity to become abnormal and possibly cancerous over time.

So how is not having a period WHILE on hormonal birth control any different? Come with me back to the bed analogy. In the previous example, the bed gets all dirty, and bugs and cats start living in it. When hormonal birth control is in play, the lining is either forced to shed regularly, OR the lining is so thin that it doesn't need to shed. Now instead of having some old nasty cat hair ridden sheets, the bed is stripped and in storage. Then when you are ready to get pregnant, you pull the bed out of storage. In the case of PCOS, you may need to make the bed and put someone in it using medication to encourage ovulation. Until that need arises, it stays wrapped in plastic and preserved while on hormonal birth control. That's why you don't need to bleed.

Clomiphene citrate is a medication used sometimes to encourage ovulation. Metformin (yes, the medication used to manage diabetes), can be used to aid in ovulation and weight loss. There are also herbal medications that can be used to encourage ovulation like Myoinositol. Sometimes more intense fertility treatments are needed. The diagnosis of PCOS is complicated. It is based on a constellation of symptoms and findings that I cannot bring myself to delve into in this chapter. Suffice it to say, irregularly or infrequent menstrual cycles, weight gain, and excessive facial or body hair growth are reasons to see your gynecologist for more evaluation. My rule of thumb is that a person should not go any longer than two months between periods if they are not on regular hormonal birth control. Even if you don't want hormonal birth control, at least have a progesterone withdrawal bleed every two months. Change those sheets.

Polyps

Polyps are also known as useless troublemakers. A polyp is like that neighbor who doesn't contribute anything positive to your life but just shares all of their personal and peripheral gossip whenever you see them. Nothing positive comes from the discussion, and if anything, you walk away feeling icky and drained. Like that character from In Living Color played by Kim Wayans. "You haven't heard it from me." How is that lady like a polyp? Well, polyps grow for no good reason. They are there just because, which is not a reason, and all they do is cause prolonged, heavy or irregular bleeding.

Polyps are like skin tags in that they come out of nowhere and often for no reason. Why do they bleed? Normally blood loss is controlled by the constriction of the muscles around blood vessels. Imagine a water hose that has a sheath that narrows by itself to shut off the water. That hose could stop water from being lost. Polyps don't contain muscle, so the blood vessels don't close off as easily and a woman is more likely to bleed. The other way that polyps cause trouble is that, like fibroids, polyps can block the area in the uterus that a pregnancy would want to implant. It's like if you just did laundry and clean clothes are all over your bed, but you want to go to sleep. You are probably going to have to either put the clothes away or sweep them all onto the floor to make room to lie down. Likewise, to allow for pregnancy in the setting of an intracavitary polyp, the polyp often needs to be removed to clear the bed.

Polyps really don't usually appear as a result of something their landlord did. The exception to that rule is someone who is overweight with abnormal menstruation. These women can sometimes grow uterine lining so irregularly that polyps are more likely to form. Another scenario that is pro-polyp formation is when a woman is on Tamoxifen therapy post-breast cancer treatment.

So, what can be done? First, if a polyp is not causing symptoms of heavy or irregular bleeding, it doesn't always need to be removed. Sometimes polyps are discovered incidentally during ultrasound for another purpose. Like fibroids, if they don't bother you, they usually don't bother me. I just monitor to ensure that size and contour are stable as long as a woman is at low risk for developing cancer. If necessary, polyps can be removed hysteroscopically. See Hysteroscopy for more about that procedure. Hormonal birth control is often good at controlling overgrowth of the uterine lining. That includes oral contraceptives and progestin-containing IUDs (LN-IUD). As with everything, I would defer to the judgment and recommendations of your own doctor. Why? Because they know YOU—your symptoms, your history, and your testing so far. That is how Dr. Google will steer you wrong. It will give you 101 ways to die, but not factor in YOUR story.

Popcorn

Forgive the redundancy if you read my opening to the A Section. I have been waiting for this moment for so long. I had been conceptualizing and writing other books for years, though I never finished any of them. On that fateful day when my wonderful patient told me that her vagina smelled like popcorn, I involuntarily chuckled. I was not trying to be a jerk, I was genuinely amused and couldn't hold it in. It was a Gyne Blooper Reel moment. She then proceeds to tell me that "popcorn smell of the vagina is a thing." No, really. She Googled it and so many women complained of this. Well, I proceeded to evaluate her situation and didn't actually find anything wrong with her, but I did go to Google later. No, not for education but for sheer entertainment.

I discovered pages upon pages of posts and articles about this subject. Buttered popcorn, not buttered, "I eat a lot of popcorn", "I never eat popcorn", folks with their pubic hair cut in the image of Orville Redenbacher, and the list went on and on. #slightexaggerationwiththatlastone

If you came to this section to find out WHY these women's lady parts smelled like the box office on opening day, I'll have more for you in the SMELL section. Women have told me that their discharge smelled like cinnamon, swamp water, and a variety of other both pleasant and unpleasant smells. I treat them all like I treat most things in medicine:

- I listen to the person's full story—we call this "taking their history"
- I perform a physical exam—checking them out with my senses of sight, touch, and sometimes inadvertently, my sense of smell
- I check laboratory tests when indicated—A swab can test for a lot of things including sexually transmitted infections, bacterial overgrowth, yeast infections, etc.

Sometimes I can solve the problem like I'm playing a weird game of Clue, without a candlestick. Sometimes if I can't find a cause and the symptoms resolve on their own, I chalk it up to a diagnosis that I named years ago: Periodic Weirdness. My personal, non-evidence based theory is that every woman is entitled to have something weird happen to her or come from within her every once in a while, whether physically or emotionally. As long as it is infrequent, mild, and resolves itself, I can concede that I don't ALWAYS have the answers. Don't tell my husband that. (I'm sure he already knows.)

One of my favorite comedians Dave Helem once mentioned in a routine that a vagina that he once knew smelled like scallops. (I'll take popcorn over shellfish any day!)

Postpartum Depression

In Season 4, Episode 2 of Blackish, Bow went through postpartum depression after the delivery of their fifth child. They showed her sadness, anxiety and deep emotional turmoil so vividly that it brought mothers that I know to tears. I too, in retrospect, think that I experienced this syndrome with at least one if not all of my pregnancies. Mine didn't display itself as overt sadness, aimless crying or physical pain. Mine was rage. I was pissed, at my husband mostly. I don't recall the details, but he does.

The Postpartum Depression Alliance of Illinois has a great summary of symptoms that women may experience:
A mother may:
- Feel constantly tired
- Feel angry, irritable or short-tempered
- Cry often for no apparent reason
- Feel panicky
- Worry excessively about her own or the baby's health

- Have a lack of feeling for the baby
- Have difficulty sleeping or eating
- Have problems concentrating
- Have frightening thoughts or fantasies
- Feel an overwhelming sense of loss

Women may say things like:

- I feel like running away.
- I don't feel like myself anymore.
- I'm a bad person, a bad mother.
- I feel like I'm going crazy!
- I sometimes think of hurting the baby or myself.

A partner may say:

- I never know what to expect when I get home
- Will my partner ever be the same?
- Something is horribly wrong, but I don't know how to help her.
- It's tough to live with a depressed person.

Depending on the severity of a woman's symptoms, she may be able to get some sleep, talk it out with family or go for a walk and feel better. Another may need to see her doctor, talk with a therapist (psychologist or psychiatrist), possibly take antidepressants temporarily, or in some circumstances, be hospitalized. The point is women and families should not be ashamed if these symptoms arise. Recognizing them can help protect relationships and make new motherhood way more enjoyable.

And what about eating or encapsulating the placenta? More data needs to be collected to determine if there is any value, but data analysis thus far is not demonstrating a reproducible or consistent benefit to new mothers. As with any bodily fluid or tissue, there are risks to consumption that should also be fully explored. There is not a standard form of processing that a practitioner can be held to. That's like eating food from a new Mom & Pop food truck that doesn't have a food service license. The food may be delicious, but if they don't have a license, you don't know if their behind-the-scenes food handling won't poison you one day. To be put simply, at this point I cannot recommend placental encapsulation because of safety concerns and the lack of consistent data supporting a benefit. Eat placenta at your own risk.

Pregnancy

Hopefully, you have already learned a lot about pregnancy from the Contraception, Fertility and Labor sections. I'd like to break THIS section up into desired vs. undesired pregnancy and touch on some need-to-know topics before trying to conceive called "preconception counseling."

I'm Not "Trying":

To recap some basic pregnancy truths, it takes one sexual encounter involving egg and sperm to lead to pregnancy, even though every sexual encounter may not lead to pregnancy. Knowing that truth is important. People will tell me they don't need to use birth control or condoms because they don't have sex "that much". Sex and pregnancy are not dose dependent. Things that are dose dependent are like alcohol consumption. If you drink too much for too long, you will end up having liver disease. If you eat too much for too long without adequate exercise, you will end up with excess weight and heart problems among other things.

Sex is not like that. Sure the more times you have sex, the more likely you are to eventually get pregnant, but it only takes once. Flip a coin and it will land or heads or tails. The more you flip, the more of each result, but getting heads could easily only take one flip. Think of sex like playing dice, except the dice have only three sides rather than six. Each time you have sex, you roll, and 30% of the time you will land on pregnancy. Expand this analogy out to a year of rolling. About 90% of people will be pregnant after 1 year of unprotected intercourse. Use an uncertain method like rhythm or pull out, 20% will be pregnant after one year. Use condoms inconsistently, or consider the failure rate of dysfunctional condoms, and still, you are at 20% failure rate. IUDs are 99% effective, which is why I've said it before, and I'll say it again: They are my favorite.

To the people who tell me that they are not trying but are not using any form of birth control, I say this: If you are not actively preventing pregnancy, by OB/GYN calculations, you ARE trying. You should be as prepared as possible to get pregnant or to be pregnant if/when it happens. Take prenatal vitamins, or at least a multivitamin, be mindful of the medications you are taking, if any, and their safety in pregnancy, track your periods so that you know if you missed one, and so on. Behave as though you are...

"Trying":

If you desire and are pursuing pregnancy before it actually

occurs, you are now entering the realm where you could benefit from pre-conception counseling. I individualize preconception consults based on my patient's medical history. There are general principles though, that I can divulge. I break this discussion into two parts— the "how do I try to get pregnant" (aside from the obvious) and the "how should I prepare myself for being pregnant." The recommendations that fall into my "how to try" category are the following:

• Download a period tracking app, preferably a free one. These make it easier to know if your menstrual cycles are regular, as well as the first day of your last menstrual period when you get that positive test. I don't think women need to start with ovulation sticks or fancy wrist bands only because in my experience they increase anxiety, are sometimes pricey, and are often unnecessary. To each her own though.

• Have sex, vaginal intercourse that is, at least every other day around the projected time of ovulation. No need to do "it" more often than once per day, just so the man has an opportunity to create a good quantity of solid sperm. I specified vaginal intercourse because I have had a handful of experiences where the couple didn't realize that anal sex wouldn't get you pregnant. You think I'm lying…

• A woman should be on prenatal vitamins ideally before she tries. This sets her up with a good reservoir of iron, calcium, folic acid, etc. If she isn't on vitamins prior to conception, that isn't a recipe for disaster, but it is just better if she is. The man can often also benefit from a healthy diet with antioxidants like green leafy vegetables. No laptop use on his lap, encouraging loose underwear, and eliminating hot tub soaking, due to the effects of higher temperature on semen quality, can help as well.

• If you are under 35, give it up to one year to conceive. Each month, there is only about a 30% chance of conceiving, but about 90% of women will be pregnant after 1 year of unprotected intercourse. If you are 35 or over, we generally advise trying for 6 months before seeking further evaluation and assistance in trying to get pregnant. This is not to say that there has to be something wrong if it takes longer than 6 months, but time is of the essence so you don't want to waste it if there is something wrong.

• If we do get to 12 months, or 6 months (35 or older), and there is no baby in the uterus, we need to be prepared to check the uterine structure with an ultrasound, make sure the tubes are opened, check some hormone levels including a thyroid test, and we can't leave out the fellas, so we check a semen analysis. Meanwhile, I advise my patients to make an appointment to see a specialist in reproductive endocrinology and infertility (REI). I can start the work-up, but whether or not I find a cause, we still need to get her a baby.

On to the "be as prepared to be pregnant as possible" topic:
- Regular exercise is recommended pre-pregnancy. That's 150 minutes of light to moderate exercise per week, or intense exercise 75 minutes per week. That sounds like a lot, but if you do 30 minutes of moderate cardio 5-days per week, you're there. I don't mind the cross-fitters of the world doing their cross fit thing up until the pregnancy test is positive. Once it is positive, though, stepping back the intensity to 75-80% of your usual is recommended to decrease miscarriage risk. Being at a healthy weight pre-pregnancy is ideal for improving fertility and reduction of risks within pregnancy. Overweight and obese women are more likely to develop diabetes in pregnancy, high blood pressure, and even disorders like preeclampsia.
- Alcohol, caffeine, and other drugs: I don't mind it if you drink alcohol up until the positive test, but if you are in the timeframe post ovulation where you could be pregnant, maybe stick with no more than 2 drinks in a sitting. Once the pregnancy is declared, say no to alcohol. Caffeine falls into my "less is more" category. I would love for my ladies to be off of caffeine in pregnancy, but even I needed a boost here and there. The max recommended amount is 2 cups of regular strength coffee per day, which should equate to 200mg of caffeine. Staying below this number should not increase your miscarriage risk. In extreme circumstances, excessive caffeine can increase stillbirth risk. Go decaf if you really need a little somethin' somethin'. Smoking, marijuana and other illicit drugs are a definite no during pregnancy. Nothing good can come from exposing these developing cells that are forming a human to those toxins. This includes second-hand smoke. Also remember, that risk of SIDS (sudden infant death syndrome), asthma and other ailments go up in households where smoking occurs, even if not directly around the baby.
- Genetic testing is available if interested to determine if you or the father carry any genetic diseases that could be passed to the

baby and cause disease. The difference between a carrier and a person who has a disease is that the carrier has just the building blocks or puzzle pieces for the disease but not the actual disease. Imagine if two people had the perfectly matched puzzle pieces that fit together just right, they could have a baby affected by whatever was on their puzzle. Genetic testing is now available through the blood to check couples for these carrier traits. A common disease that requires two "puzzle" pieces is sickle cell trait/disease. Another one is cystic fibrosis. This testing is completely optional, but it can give couples the heads up if they may need to become a little more specific about how they try to conceive—possibly using advanced conception methods to avoid having a baby with a debilitating disease.

This is the abbreviated version of a preconception consult. Make an appointment to discuss issues and recommendations that are specific to you. Lastly, the CYA in me doesn't want to tell you what meds you can safely take in pregnancy because I don't know you. I can contribute a sample list of medication that you should NOT take without discussing with your doctor first. Some medications include certain types of blood pressure medication, ibuprofen, naproxen, aspirin, certain acne medications, certain types of antibiotics, and stimulant laxatives among others. Thyroid medication and diabetic medications often need significant adjustments in early pregnancy. Speak to your doctor right away if you are on any of these meds. Okay, okay, I'll give you a few benign meds that you can take for nausea since that often hits first:

- Ginger
- Pepcid (famotidine)—since reflux and nausea often go hand in hand
- Vitamin B6 three times a day
- Doxylamine (found in Unisom sleep tabs)

Premenstrual Syndrome- PMS

Premenstrual Syndrome, or PMS, is that resting bitch face, or RBF, that lives within you, that comes out before your period. That same chick comes out of me when I'm tired. In fact, I think that the real me actually takes a nap when I'm tired and RBF, or Ribfy, as I like to call her (actually, I never called her that until this exact moment), takes over. That children's movie Inside Out characterized it perfectly. Except, in me, instead of Joy, Disgust,

Sadness, Anger, and Fear, it's me and Ribfy when I am post-call. She starts every sentence in my head with "Do Better" and end's every statement with "I have nothing for you". My medical assistant used to abbreviate my classic phrase by saying, "IHNFY," because "I have nothing for you" summarized that moment when we had nothing left to give and YOU would just have to figure it out.

Ironically, as close as Ribfy and I are, I don't think I have personally experienced PMS. This could be because I choose to not have periods. I did get the angry and annoyed version of postpartum depression. I can only imagine that PMS is on that scale.

According to the National Institute of Health, Premenstrual Syndrome is a set of physical and psychological symptoms that usually start about 7 to 10 days before a woman gets her monthly period (menstrual cycle). The symptoms are not just emotional. Many women experience breast tenderness, headaches, back pain, and joint or muscle aches. They may also have water retention, bloating, and sleeping problems or digestive problems.

Women who have PMS often feel exhausted, down, irritable and have lower self-esteem in the days leading up to their period. Women might feel like they are losing control over their body and emotions. For some, PMS can be improved with birth control. For others, different birth control options can make it worse. Counseling is an option. Never underestimate the power of a good psychologist or psychiatrist. Anti-depressants are also an option. Anti-depressants can be taken daily or just for 10-14 days leading up to the period. The first step is recognition of the problem.

Severe premenstrual symptoms can actually become premenstrual dysphoric disorder, or PMDD. Like PMS, premenstrual dysphoric disorder follows a predictable, cyclic pattern. The symptoms of PMDD are more severe than those seen with PMS, but in most cases, the symptoms still stop when, or shortly after, the period begins. If your version of Ribfy is messing with your life or friendships/relationships, you may need some help. Regular exercise, yoga and meditation, and if needed, medical intervention can often improve symptoms. Don't be ashamed. We know that the "real" you is actually nice (right?).

Probiotics

Probiotics are "good" bacteria. I know that you germaphobes out there must be thinking, "That sounds like an oxymoron." Well, there are bacteria that work with our bodies to keep us healthy. The best examples are the bacteria in our intestines and the bacteria in the vagina. The bacteria in our intestines help us digest foods, regulate which components of the food we need to absorb, and manage waste we don't need. Yes, the bacteria in your funky dirty feces is there for a reason. I know you like to think your $#!+ don't stink, but lean a little bit closer and see that roses really smell like boo boo boo. #thelovebelow #andre3000 #hashtagsstilldontworkinbooks

There are certain bacteria that live and prosper in the vagina. The problem with consuming oral probiotics is that we don't really know how bacteria make it to our vaginas through our digestive systems. I would love to say all vaginas would remain in perfect balance if they were regularly dosed with healthy bacteria pills or drinks. Like if you apply fertilizer to the garden, all of the flowers should bloom. Unfortunately, neither the vagina nor your garden is quite that predictable. (Remember, I have the anti-green thumb.)

There are some probiotics that have legitimate evidence of being effective in repopulating the vagina with normal bacteria. Two that are seen repeatedly in the literature are L. rhamnosus and L. fermentum, later renamed L. reuteri.

From the Oxford Journal:

"Probiotics, especially L. acidophilus, L. rhamnosus GR-1 and L. fermentum (reuteri)RC-14, may be considered as potential empirical preventive agents in women who suffer from frequent episodes of VVC [Vulvovaginal candidiasis] (more than three episodes per year) since adverse effects from their use are scarce..."

From the NIH:

"L. rhamnosus GR-1 and L. reuteri RC-14 probiotic group [led to more] lactobacilli-dominated normal vaginal microbiota restored from a BV [bacterial vaginosis] vaginal flora..."

Translation: Those two bacteria when consumed seemed to reset the normal balance of vagina bacteria and decrease the frequency of yeast and bacterial vaginosis. I still drink a Kombucha every now and then and take a probiotic if it is within arms-reach, especially if it has those two bacteria in it. There isn't evidence of harm that I am aware of, so why not take it if it MIGHT help.

Puberty

Puberty is the time in life when a boy or girl becomes

sexually mature. It is a process that usually happens between ages 10 and 14 for girls and ages 12 and 16 for boys. It causes physical changes and affects boys and girls differently. In girls, the first sign of puberty is usually breast development. Thank you, MedlinePlus.gov.

Let's be honest, you have as much access to Google as I do. What you want from me is the stuff that is too cryptic or boring on Google. Let's talk about, "when keeping it real [pubescent] goes wrong." #comedycentral #davechappelle. How early is too early? How late is too late?

It is normal for puberty to begin any time between the ages of 8 and 14. The presence of hair under the arms and in the pubic area in addition to the formation of breast buds signify the beginning of this stage in a girl's life. Within months to years, she will also start having periods, no more than two years after the aforementioned signs of puberty. If the period doesn't start by the two-year mark after breasts and hair arrive, you should see a doctor. If you need one more sign that puberty is coming, I'm told that one of the best signs in girls is the conversion of "little sweet precious" girl, to "BEEEAAATTTTCH." I must have never gone through puberty then (side-eye to myself).

The lack of a period can be a sign of a hormonal or genetic issue. Too long or aggressive periods can be a sign of, well, being a girl. Okay, sometimes there is a problem there too, but often there isn't anything wrong with girls with aggressive periods. Periods suck, especially in puberty. Often to improve the situation, regular exercise and weight loss in the overweight teen can help. In the extremely active normal or underweight teen, periods can be few and far between because of the activity level and physical stress that it causes. Eating disorders can do this too. Weight gain or psychotherapy should be tried when appropriate. Hormonal birth control can also be considered for cycle control—including decreasing blood volume and pain level.

Something to consider with birth control pills and the adolescent girl is the concern for an increased frequency of developing depression and anxiety. It is not uncommon to start teenagers on birth control pills for cycle control and/or birth control, but being aware of this possible side effect can help us to know if she may need to be switched to a different birth control method.

The take-home points: Puberty in girls should occur between the ages of 8 and 14 and should begin with underarm and pubic hair and breast buds, then culminate in blood and attitude (that last one only in some cases). If this sequence of events doesn't happen in that time frame, your pediatrician or gynecologist can help navigate the "what's happening" space.

Pull-Out

See the Men Section, SMH. #dreverywoman #iwroteasongaboutit

Q.

Questions

Some of my favorite questions are truly the inspiration for this entire literary work. I answer questions constantly that are more common than women would think because these topics don't get discussed amongst friends. Here are a few of my favorites. I am literally asking for a friend:

Q: What are genital warts and how common are they?
A: Genital warts are skin growth caused by the HPV virus. They can mimic the appearance of skin tags or grow to look like cauliflower on your skin. More on what "things" can be in the genital region in the Things Explained section.

Q: Is bowel urgency common after having a baby?
A: Anything goes after having a baby. Some women find themselves with urinary urgency or incontinence, meaning going to the washroom to urinate becomes a right-now thing and sometimes you don't make it before the golden shower rains down. Fecal urgency and incontinence are also a possibility, especially depending on the severity of the tear during delivery. I say give it at least 6 weeks to 3 months to resolve. If symptoms are improving in that time frame, see it through. If they don't improve within that time frame or are not resolved by the 3-month mark, it is important to follow up with your gynecologist to see what the next step may be.

Q: How long is too long to not have a period?
A: If you are on hormonal birth control, be it a pill, patch, ring, shot or hormonal IUD, I am fine with you never having a period at all. Periods are optional. If you are not on hormonal birth control, I don't like ladies to go more than 2 months without a period. I dissected this topic in the Menstrual Cycle section. I'll summarize it again here.

When on hormonal birth control (the copper IUD or condoms don't count), the uterine lining is thinned to the point of not bleeding. It's like having a yard. The shorter the grass is, the fewer clippings there will be if you mow it. If you mow a lawn that is just concrete with no grass, there will be no clippings at all. That is the state of a uterus on low estrogen birth control. The uterine lining grows in response to more estrogen. IF the birth control is pro-progesterone or low estrogen, the uterine lining thins and nothing will come out when your "period" is signaled.

If your uterus is not subjected to hormonal birth control, but you are not having regular periods, the lining grows and grows and grows, but never sheds. This is caused by unopposed estrogen. The uterine lining overgrowth is like a yard that is unattended. The grass gets all crazy and out of control and weeds begin to grow and take over. Similarly, that unshed lining can become abnormal, and possibly precancerous or cancerous. This lining needs to shed periodically, just like your lawn needs to be mowed periodically. Hormonal birth control controls the uterine landscaping, which is why periods are optional.

Q: How common is Herpes?
A: Very. Here is a genital herpes chart from MMWR.

Source: Xu F, Sternberg MR, Gottlieb SL, Berman SM, Markowitz LE, Forhan SE, Taylor (23 April 2010). "Seroprevalence of Herpes Simplex Virus Type 2 Among Persons Aged 14–49 Years—United States, 2005–2013". Morbidity and Mortality

Demographic	HSV-2 Seroprevalence	(Females)	(Males)
Gender	16.2%	20.9%	11.5%
Age: 14–19 yrs	1.4%	2.1%	0.8%
Age: 20–29 yrs	10.5%	14.4%	6.6%
Age: 30–39 yrs	19.6%	25.2%	13.9%
Age: 40–49 yrs	26.1%	32.3%	19.6%
Ethnicity: White, non-Hispanic	12.3%	15.9%	8.7%
Ethnicity: Black, non-Hispanic	39.2%	48.0%	29.0%
Ethnicity: Mexican American	10.1%	13.2%	7.5%
1 Lifetime Sex Partner	3.9%	5.4%	1.7%
2–4 Lifetime Sex Partners	14.0%	18.8%	7.3%
5–9 Lifetime Sex Partners	16.3%	21.8%	10.1%
>10 Lifetime Sex Partners	26.7%	37.1%	19.1%

Weekly Report (MMWR). **59** (15): 456–459. PMID 20414188. Retrieved 12 April 2011.

Source: Xu F, Sternberg MR, Gottlieb SL, Berman SM, Markowitz LE, Forhan SE, Taylor (23 April 2010). "Seroprevalence of Herpes Simplex Virus Type 2 Among Persons Aged 14–49 Years—United States, 2005–2013". Morbidity and Mortality Weekly Report (MMWR). 59 (15): 456–459. PMID 20414188. Retrieved 12 April 2011.

Though genital herpes is commonly caused by HSV 2, it can be caused by HSV 1. Both cause the same symptoms, but they behave differently when it comes to their frequency of recurrence and extent of lesions. HSV 1 is commonly the cause of oral and nasal cold sores. I went over that more comprehensively in the Cold Sore section.

Q: How do I make sure that when I get pregnant, I am going to have a boy or a girl?

A: Well, when the moon is in the third orbit, and the bed faces east, and the Chinese calendar shows that it is the year of a chicken, and you have your right leg up at a 60 degree angle, YOU will be certain to have a blessed baby if the Lord says the same. Whether it is a boy or girl, I can't say. If I could help you to be certain about gender with "natural" conception, I would be super rich. With in vitro fertilization, or IVF, this is a little different. There is this thing called pre-implantation genetics where the egg and sperm are fertilized in a laboratory, and the embryo is allowed to grow for a little while. Then a single cell is taken from each embryo and tested for certain chromosomes, which can include sex chromosomes. This process is usually used to try to avoid severe diseases that are carried by the parents. Then the one or two embryos with the ideal genes are placed back into the uterus to hopefully grow.

With typical skin-on-skin conception, the sex determination comes from the man, who contributes either an X or a Y chromosome within each sperm. That X or Y is what determines the sex. Mom can only give X's since a woman is generally XX herself. That means that if the sperm has an X, a female will be created. If it has a Y, then you'll have a male. XX = girl. XY = boy. Gender discussions aside, I am just talking penis vs. vagina.

This seems like the perfect time to bring up chromosomal abnormalities. When I see a future mom or a couple who is disappointed about the sex of their gestating baby, I get a little frustrated, only because a healthy baby is a blessing not to be taken for granted. My bias is that I have seen a lot of babies born, sometimes living and sometimes stillborn. I have seen a wide array of abnormalities from Down Syndrome (yes, it is Down, not Down's), to abdominal wall defects, to even sex chromosome and hormone abnormalities resulting in ambiguous genitalia. Translation: when the baby was born, we didn't know if it was a boy or a girl. My soap-box point is that I believe anyone really should be happy with any baby, especially if the baby is healthy.

Q: Why do yeast infections and urinary tract infections happen?
A: Your guess is as good as mine. Mostly these infections arise spontaneously, but I do go into more depth in the UTI and Candida sections regarding how to try to avoid them.

Q: What is the difference between vaginal infections and urinary tract infections?

A: More on this in the UTI section, but the summary is that the urethra is where you urinate. Your vagina is where you vaginate. Just kidding. The vagina and the urethra are two separate holes. The vagina has a lot of bacteria in it normally, kind of like the mouth. The urethra, despite being down there only a couple of short centimeters away, is sterile. It is bacteria--free. The bladder and kidneys hate bacteria. Here they are, though, the unwilling neighbors of the vagina and, down the hall, the rectum. Dorm Vulva is where Ms. Urethra, Vagina and Rectum all live. If they keep to themselves, Uree can keep her room clean and not be bothered by Vag and Rec. If the trash from Vag or Rec gets swept in the wrong direction, Uree can find herself with a dirty floor and ants. If the situation gets out of hand, Antibiotic Dorm mother needs to come in and help Urethra. As voluntary as my analogy seems, most of the time we really cannot control the frequency of UTIs. Wiping from front to back and urinating after sex can help. Overall good health and immune system strength are a must.

Q: Is it normal to have painful periods? Is taking birth control to control the pain and heavy bleeding just masking the underlying symptoms?

A: Yes, periods suck. Of course, there are always extremes. Cramping and pain that is so debilitating that it results in time off of work or school, causes nausea and vomiting or is not relieved by the bottle-dose acetaminophen or ibuprofen regimen, may not be normal. See your doctor for evaluation and pain relief options. Often in my adolescent patients, depending on their symptoms, I try to get their pain under control with pain medication or by using birth control. Birth control side effects should be monitored closely in adolescents because depression can be more common in this population.

I usually only call on the power of ultrasound if the initial symptom management is either unsuccessful or laden with too many unwanted side effects. Ultrasound can sometimes point to the cause, but sometimes it doesn't and the procedure itself can be uncomfortable. If an ultrasound is performed but doesn't show any abnormality, I begin to suspect endometriosis. Endometriosis is the Keyser Soze of the pelvis—see the Endometriosis section for more about that. The point is that the diagnosis of endometriosis is not always easy to make, thus the success of the treatment is sometimes what we use to guide our conclusion about the diagnosis. If the treatment works, great. If it doesn't, we need to look for another diagnosis.

Q: Is an IUD going to kill me?
A: If it is, I need to say my goodbyes now. If it is, then I have been on death's doorstep for years. If it is, I should be ashamed about how many that I place regularly. But wait, are my ladies dropping like flies? No. Most, as in 9 out of 10 women, love their IUD. The vast majority of IUDs that I remove are removed because the ladies are ready to conceive. It is rare that I remove one for dissatisfaction or impending doom. More on IUDs in the Contraceptive section.

R.

Remember that show from the early '90s on Nickelodeon Roundhouse?
The theme song said, "We'll have a celebration, where I can be myself. Whenever my life gets me so down I know I can go down, to where the music and the fun never end. As long as the music keeps playing I know what I'm saying. I know that I can find a friend... down at the Roundhouse."
Why am I bringing this up? Well, R is stumping me a little in this exact moment, but what I loved about that show is that it was so different, and it celebrated comedy and entertainment by and for young people. I thought that I could have been a cast member on that show. It introduced me to people who were confident and seemed larger than life even before being grown-ups. #ireminisce #powerfulnia
Wait, I just thought of a women's health R. It's not a fun one though.

Rape
Defined by my girl Merriam (I explained our relationship back in the Feminism section) as: "unlawful sexual activity and

usually sexual intercourse carried out forcibly or under threat of injury against the will, usually of a female or with a person who is beneath a certain age or incapable of valid consent."

Anywhere from 80-90% of rape or sexual assault victims know their attacker. Sexual assault is NEVER the victim's fault. If you are sexually assaulted, please go to the emergency room right away. Going to the emergency department means that you are examined for any infections (which you should repeat again in 6 months), and it also creates a paper trail that can be used to support what you are saying happened. If you have medical documentation, it can carry as much weight as a police report, which you should file as well. If you are hesitant because you are embarrassed or ashamed or just don't want to relive or stay in the incident, my only piece of advice is for you to think of the next victim. You likely were not the first person this happened to with this person. If you don't want them to do it again, make them face.

8
SEX: BETWEEN THE SHEETS
OF PAPER

S.

Sex

CNN recently released an article about why Americans are having less sex. The article proposed multiple reasons, including the increased phone and social media distraction. One of my favorite quotes from the article, (because it is interesting, not because I can relate in any way, fyi, btw, ijs, tmi), was from psychologist Margie Nichols:

Compared with earlier generations, women might be viewing sex as less of a duty to their husbands and more of a personal choice. "It makes sense that women in relationships might be losing their sex drive and saying 'no' more, as opposed to my mother's generation that just spread their legs and composed a shopping list in their heads during sex," she said. "If that's true, then the decline in frequency is a good thing."

A middle-aged patient once told me, "There is a big difference between doing it and enjoying it." She gave me permission to quote her, as do all of my ladies whose examples I've used in this book. She was speaking in reference to her recent decision to not have sex anymore because of pain/discomfort for which I was helping to treat her. This discrepancy between "doing it and enjoying it" was painfully clear to her.

Sometimes the disconnect between her desire and his is related to pain or discomfort. Sometimes it is an issue of interest due to issues external to the relationship. Sometimes the issues are within the relationship. Sometimes they are both perfectly happy with one another, but the disconnect arises between how often he wants to and how often SHE WANTS to. Once a month, once a week, or once a day can ALL be considered too often or too infrequent depending on who I'm talking to.

My job is to help the woman understand if her feelings are reasonable by normalizing them when they are common. I also encourage her to communicate said feelings with her significant other rather than just with me. Sex therapy is also a "thing" and there are even meds now available to help women increase interest.

Then there is a common scenario where the precedence of sexual frequency and enthusiasm set in the "courting" stage falls off of a cliff when marriage and KIDS come into the picture. I personally know of a number of couples who didn't have sex at all before they got married, so the aftermath was, by my calculations, the come up (no pun intended). If two people start off getting "it in" (or getting "it on" depending on how cool you are with your phraseology) every day, then over time go to once per week or once per month because of life and kids, I could see one or both partners feeling some kind of way about that. The remedy? I don't know. Don't set the bar so high? Spend some quality time with your spouse? Talk to the Lord? The latter two always work well for me.

Sexually Transmitted Diseases

I almost never call someone to tell them they have a sexually transmitted disease and hear the response, "Oh I know. I figured that I had that." With rare exception, most of my ladies do not feel symptoms or have any indication that would lead them to expect a test to be positive. STDs are on the rise. Per the Center for Disease Control, "Total combined cases of chlamydia, gonorrhea, and syphilis reported in 2015 reached the highest number ever."

Some ladies routinely decline STD testing. I offer testing to everyone every year. Married, single, engaged, it doesn't matter. I am going to offer testing. I think that women are sometimes afraid to test, and others believe it is a disrespectful act that indicates distrust of their partner. I think that periodic STD testing is responsible and keeps all parties safe. I am a little biased because I see a lot of unexpected results.

What about this little bomb—coming up positive for an STD doesn't always equate to infidelity. I knew a man who found out years into marriage that his wife had HIV. She wasn't cheating; she just hadn't been tested in a decade. She found out incidentally in blood tests during a physical. They are still married, by the way. That's LOVE.

So who NEEDS to be tested? As I stated, anyone can be tested for STDs every year or as needed, but some are at higher risk than others, like anyone with a new sexual partner. These are the ladies who sound like nails on a chalkboard to me if they decline testing. Even if a partner says he has been tested, do you know when this testing was done relative to his most recent sexual encounter, and for what he was tested? There is not a universal "STD test." Specific things have to be checked. Here are some basic fun STD facts from the Center for Disease Control:

Gonorrhea/Chlamydia: According to the CDC 2015 stats (2016 has not been reported at the time of this book), "Americans ages 15 to 24 years old accounted for nearly two-thirds of chlamydia diagnoses and half of gonorrhea diagnoses".

Trichomoniasis: "Most women found to have Trichomoniasis (85%) reported no symptoms…Prevalence of Trichomoniasis increases with age and lifetime number of sexual partners…"

HIV: "If we look at HIV diagnoses by race and ethnicity, we see that African Americans are most affected by HIV. In 2015, African Americans made up only 13% of the US population but had 45% of all new HIV diagnoses. Additionally, Hispanic/Latinos are also strongly affected. They made up 18% of the US population but had 24% of all new HIV diagnoses."

Syphilis: "Women's rate of syphilis diagnosis increased by more than 27 percent from 2014 to 2015" (CDC).

Herpes: "Herpes simplex virus (HSV) is among the most prevalent of sexually transmitted infections." Blood testing for HSV 2 is reportedly as common as 15% to 52% of women, depending on their ethnicity. Evidence of disease is not always directly correlated with positive blood testing. This one is complicated to diagnose, but honestly, it is one of the most benign STDs from a danger-to-your-body standpoint. That said, since you can never rid yourself completely of it, it is best to avoid this diagnosis.

STD testing is not automatically performed at all doctor's offices. Patients often tell me, "Oh wouldn't my internist have done testing?" I tell them, "No, not unless you asked or they specifically offered." Also keep in mind that if a partner doesn't want to use a condom, you can bet that you are probably not the exception but rather the rule. It is very possible that he (or she) infrequently uses condoms at all, which doesn't bode well for your chances of avoiding an STD (or possibly multiple).

What's the take-home message? Protect yourself and take the test, or be abstinent, which is by far the best (albeit not as common) form of prevention. There is no shame in testing; not knowing your results can hurt you and those you care about.

Sheltering

I had a patient who told me that she was raised in a culture where anatomy and sexuality weren't discussed. There was shame associated with talking about the female body, even for sheer educational purposes. I think sometimes parents shy away from discussing the body or sex because they think that more information will lead to more sexual activity. Though I don't judge people's sexual choices, it is no secret that I am a fan of abstinence and celibacy before marriage. Because of this, I have been asking women for years what drives their sexual choices when they have chosen to not have sex. It is a point of curiosity.

I can remember going away to college and being shell shocked. I saw freshmen girls from the strict households, who tasted freedom for the first time in their lives, wildin' out (that's colloquial for going crazy #urbandictionary). I witnessed real live Girls Gone Wild. You could spot a girl from a mile away who never got to date or associate with boys before college. She lost her damn mind at her first chance. I can only imagine that if these girls hadn't associated with boys before, they probably had also never had "the talk" about the "birds and the bees" or any other "air quote euphemism" like that.

In my experience, being sheltered doesn't decrease sexual activity. On the contrary, early sexual exposure that is misguided, whether by experienced yet unknowledgeable friends or inappropriate contact, isn't the recipe for healthy sexuality either. The take-home message here is information is not the enemy. Learn about and teach the next generation about their bodies. Let your example and acquisition of information help other young ladies make their own, hopefully, healthy and safe, decisions.

Sleep

The hypocrisy is that I am writing about sleep when it is presently 1:30 am. Sleep allows your body and your mind to reset. It is important for immune function, brain function, and general health. Sleep is very important, so much so that my whole family is presently doing it. Let me join them. Goodnight.

Smell

So far, I have established that you don't smell like popcorn, or if you do, I'm not sure why that is. But what do you do if you feel like you have an odor that just won't go away? The inside of the vagina can emit an odor in the setting of infection. The Vaginitis and Discharge sections tackle some of the causes of vaginal infection. But what if it isn't the inside that smells? Here are some tips to reduce external odor of the vaginal/vulva:

Get out that electric shaver and trim the hedges. Hair can hold odor so, external appearance aside, occasionally you just need to start afresh (pun intended). Electric shavers are not painful and will leave less, if any, ingrown hair or razor bumps compared to blade shavers.

Consider using stainless steel (unless you have a metal allergy!). There are stainless steel body bars that can be used in the shower that can remove odors in the same way that your stainless steel kitchen faucet can get that onion and garlic smell off of your hands. This is due to some kind of chemical reaction that I can't explain, but it works.

Use rubbing alcohol, but be careful. Bacteria on the external skin of the groin can make odors waft even after a good shower. A light application of rubbing alcohol on a cotton ball to the external skin can cut down on odors. If you aren't careful and accidentally douse the vagina itself, be ready for the burn. There is no role for using alcohol on the inside of the vagina, ever. Beware. Alcohol can also be very drying so don't do this frequently and be prepared to use an emollient moisturizer on the skin if excessive dryness occurs. Whether you think you smell like a pond or a bag of White Castle hamburgers, hopefully, these tips will help you stay fresh. Always consult your doctor if you have questions. Vaginal aroma-therapy is not a thing, so fix it.

Smoking

I am anti-tobacco in any form. Smoking cigarettes leads to lung cancer, cervical cancer, EVERY cancer, heart disease, lung disease, EVERY disease, and you just LOOK like you've lived a hard life. Just say no. #TRUTH.

What you will not get me to do is spend time in this book writing about why I don't think that we humans should smoke anything, including hookah (which is literally 100 times worse than a cigarette from a health perspective), marijuana, cigars, Black & Milds, or anything that emits smoke from something that is being actively burned or charred. Science tells us that too much charbroiled food can increase our colon cancer risk. I cannot condone intentionally putting a burning product of any type of fire in my lungs.

Auto mechanics have an increased risk of developing COPD and other lung diseases from being around a lot of auto exhaust.

The EPA had this to say about candles and incense as possible causes of indoor air pollution:

"The scientific literature review gathered information regarding the emission of various contaminants generated when burning candles and incense, as well as the potential health effects associated with exposure to these contaminants. Burning candles and incense can be sources of particulate matter. Burning candles with lead-core wicks may result in indoor air concentration of lead above EPA-recommended thresholds. Exposure to incense smoke has been linked with several illnesses, and certain brands of incense also contain chemicals suspected of causing skin irritation."

As much as I want my house to smell like the dope-est poetry set is about to start, I take information like that to heart. You will only catch me burning even a candle infrequently and in moderation.

But NOPE, I'm not going to challenge some of you all. There are a few populations that I don't mess with, and weed-smokers is one of them. I put weed-smokers right up there next to vegans and hard-core cross-fitters. You do your thing, and I'll do mine. You don't mess with me, and I won't mess with you. And no, I have never smoked ANYTHNG a day in my life.

Wait, what just happened? What if I throw in a #noshade. Better?

So Whatcha Sayin?

A song by EPMD, and a perfect introduction to this section about medical terms that are commonly misspoken. I cringe when I hear the word "conversate". If you are confused right now, you may be a person who finds yourself "conversating" from time to time. A reasonable mistake when the word stems from "conversation." I learned many years ago, however, that the actual Merriam-Webster verb is "to converse." Used in a sentence, "I would like to converse with you about that later," or "He and I conversed about that the other day." It is both a shoe and a verb (except that the accent is on the VERSE, rather than the CON).

In medicine, there are many terms that are said by patients that I don't have the heart to correct for fear of embarrassment. However, they are, well, not correct. I'm also that jerk who will let you keep talking to me and others with food stuck in your teeth. In the interest of no longer leaving my ladies with proverbial spinach in their teeth, here are a few:

Blood clog—The word is blood clot, with a T. It can refer to a dollop of blood, sometimes seen during one's period. A blood clot can also form within a person's vein and lead to breathing difficulty or leg problems. These types of blood clots can be life-threatening. People often need blood thinners after being diagnosed with an internal or venous blood clot. A family history of blood clots is also important to discuss with your doctor.

Vomic—The word is vomit, also with a T. This means to throw up. No further explanation needed.

From the pediatric division: Chicken Pops, Wingworm and Ammonia are actually Chicken Pox (pronounced pocks), Ringworm (with an R), and Pneumonia (pronounced New-mo-neea).

Mammeogram—The word is mammogram. There is no E. Just mam-O.

Colostomy—I think this one is meant to be Colonoscopy, the test to screen for colon cancer where a camera is used to look inside the bowel and remove polyps before they become cancer. Let's break this one down: Colon-Osco-Pee. Osco like the drug store.

Sugar Diabetus—Drop the sugar, literally, and just say Diabetes, pronounced Die-uh-beet-ease. Or you can just say, "I got the Shugah," and I'll smile because of the nostalgia. It's as endearing as "the gout" that my older family members complain of.

Tubalization—The procedure is tubal ligation- pronounced tubal lie-gay-shun.

Fitting that I end this section with a gynecologic term. "Fireballs in the Eucharist" is one of the original malapropisms for fibroids in the uterus. A malapropism is a fancy word that I just learned for the humorous misuse of a word. Knowing the correct word and definition can be important to your health. For example, if your mom had a blood clot in her leg in the past, you may need testing to rule out elevated risk before starting certain types of birth control. This list is only the tip of the iceberg. Don't worry though, we will be continuing this conversate-shun.

Speculum

Enter one of my favorite and most loved posts from my blog, The Gyneco-(b)Logic, is all about speculum sizes. If you haven't seen it, you're in for a treat.

I am guessing that more than the confusion about the recommended frequency of exams, more women don't see their Lady Doctor regularly because the exams are uncomfortable, even sometimes painful. Discomfort I expect. Pain, I don't.

I have been told countless times over the years that my Pap tests don't hurt. Women often marvel at how much better tolerated my exams are than with previous doctors. I don't know why that is. I have never compared my technique to other physicians'. I do want to use this moment, however, to highlight a difference in speculum sizes and types used.

In my office, we are fortunate to have speculums from all around the world. Just kidding. We actually have multiple types of speculums for different types of women. I believe that this plays a role in the tolerability of a Pap or other speculum exams.

Let's back up for a moment. The speculum is a metal or plastic device that is used to open the vagina enough to see inside. A physician can evaluate the walls of the vagina, the cervix, perform STD testing, examine discharge quality and quantity, and even perform procedures and surgeries. Speculums are necessary in the field of gynecology as a whole. What they are not is one-size-fits-all.

Enter Gyne-Bubba Gump:

You have your metal speculum, your plastic speculum, your pediatric speculum, your Graves speculum, your Pederson speculum, your disposable speculum, your reusable speculum, your bivalve speculum, your weighted speculum, your... okay enough. My blog post features pictures of all of the speculums.

The Pederson speculums are designed for women with more narrow vaginas. I prefer these for my ladies who have never had children before. The Graves are particularly useful in women who have delivered babies vaginally. The curvature allows for better visualization of the cervix.

The pediatric speculum is excellent for my patients who have not been sexually active. The population, however, that gets the most benefit from pediatric speculums is, ironically, the elderly and postmenopausal women.

If you don't like visiting your gynecologist because of the sheer weirdness of the whole experience, I can accept that sentiment. Make an appointment anyway. If you avoid this vital screening primarily because of pain, you may need a more customized evaluation. Just a thought. Oh, and one final public service announcement for complete clarification. Every speculum exam is NOT a Pap smear. An exam with the formerly (until now) dreaded speculum can be performed to visualize the cervix, to do STD testing, to evaluate abnormal bleeding, etc. The Pap smear is specifically screening for cervical cancer.

Did you know that a speculum on a bird is a feather patch, often distinctly colored, on the inner wings? Ducks have them. It's ironic that women sometimes call my speculum, duck bills. #shuckyduck #quackquack

Superstition

Yes, many of us are very superstitious as gynecologists. The writing is on the wall. What happens is when you are in OB/GYN residency, you learn that sometimes there seems to be a shift in the universe that sends everyone into labor at the exact same time. Despite the obvious inundation of birth and life, we call these moments where you are swamped with active moms laboring and delivering via all methods, of all shapes and sizes, being "killed." Just one or two ladies delivering is manageable. When the labor and delivery unit treats you like you should split yourself and become, like, three people at once, it is not always manageable. You have to check on one lady's progress before the lady with twins is ready to push, and watch the baby whose heart rate keeps dropping, hoping that the mother's cervix will make 10 centimeters before the health and safety of the baby make you offer the mother a C-section. Many a grey hair was formed on a busy L&D night.

Enter the superstition. If you walk into a labor and delivery unit and say something foolish like, "Oh, it's not too busy here. We are going to have a quiet night," then the party bus WILL pull up in front of the hospital and unload at least ten women doing old-school Lamaze he-he-hoo-hoo's in labor with diabetes and preeclampsia, and you will likely not survive the night. Instead, a simple nod and silent communication will suffice to communicate the status of the present reasonable roster of ladies and not destine you to be crushed by placentas in the next 12-24 hours.

The opposite is not true. I have no problem saying that I am about to have a rough weekend because of all of the ladies who are due. If anything, this actually may make my situation a little better because I can either expect to be super busy or be pleasantly surprised if only good and manageable things come my way. I would NEVER say, "I think it will be quiet." I am actually typing this while on call in the hospital, and I am actively hoping that even typing these examples doesn't put a hex on the rest of my call.

Ironically, I don't believe in zodiac signs, or horoscopes, or moon signs, or black cats, or broken mirrors, or stepping on cracks, or walking under ladders, or any of that stuff. I am a firm believer in the Almighty. Don't you DARE comment on my impending call day though. "Everything you done to me, gone come back to you." — Celie from the Color Purple. I thank you.

T.

Things On Your Skin

Ah, you've made it. I am speaking to my people who started in the Bump section, then went to the Lesion section. You have arrived.

I don't make a habit of referring to private places as your "thing" but for the purposes of the title and the unisex applications of this section, it works. Don't worry, I won't get graphic. Descriptive, yes, but no overly striking images of lesions will be found here. I will leave it to Google Images to show you the absolute worst case of any disease because that is what Google is good for: Making sure that you know that you could drop dead at any given moment. #ThanksGoogle

Back to the lesson at hand...
Imperfection needs inspection, so I'm 'ma let 'em understand.
From a Gyn-NE's perspective,
Every lesion has a reason. Look for classic signs and symptoms.

Sidebar: I can appreciate the fact that Snoop Dogg included contraceptive use in "Nuthin' But A 'G' Thang" back in the day. These rappers these days could take a lesson in that, 'cause ain't no lovin' good enough to get burnt while... you know the rest.

Ending that LONG parenthetic pause, sometimes even I don't know what a lesion is until I swab it or take a biopsy. There are some rules of the road that can narrow suspicion though. Ask yourself the following questions:
• Does it hurt or not?
• How long has it been there, and how long did it take to go away if it went away?
• Has it changed in appearance or color, or multiplied?
• Are you sexually active, especially unprotected, and especially with a new partner? (Remember that things can be transmitted even if you have had the same partner for a long time

and use condoms consistently.)
• Is your groin sore/are lymph nodes swollen and tender right in that crease between your legs and your pubic region?

I am going to try to break down the top 10 causes of lesions and their characteristics in a systematic way to help you know how concerned you need to be or how far out you can chill. Get out your handheld mirror and let's get started.

Folliculitis/Hidradenitis Suppurativa

These are ingrown hairs and infected hair follicles and sweat glands, classically known as boils. If you have course curly hair, shaving can increase your risk for developing ingrown hairs. If you are prone to having ingrown hairs, you may need to use an electric hair clipper rather than a razor in order to not cut the hair beneath the skin. Electric clippers don't leave your skin super smooth, but you have to choose which is worst: Stubble, or numerous puss-filled painful bumps. Being overweight can also increase your risk of developing infected sweat glands that will classically grow and cause pain, prior to rupture. Weight loss can decrease their frequency and severity. Treat by applying warm compresses twice daily and warm baths. If that doesn't help, you may need to have them drained by a doctor. Put the needle away, lady. Occasionally I have women use topical or oral antibiotics as well. Let your doctor make that call.

Skin Tag

Skin tags are fleshy, not painful, small growths that usually appear slowly, and then just stay. They don't usually enlarge over time, but a person can develop multiple tags, much like a person can develop multiple moles over time. Skin tags aren't dangerous but can sometimes be annoying if they get caught in clothing or jewelry. There is nothing wrong with showing them to your doctor to make sure that's what they are. Biopsies are not unreasonable to confirm the diagnosis if it is unclear. Often that is not needed for a skin tag.

Genital Warts

Genital warts are caused by the HPV virus and are sexually transmitted. They are painless and grow slowly, but multiply more rapidly than skin tags. They may even grow on top of each other like broccoli or cauliflower. They are flesh colored but often slightly harder in texture than skin tags. They are not always easy to distinguish from molluscum (that's next) even by a trained eye. This is where biopsies come back into the conversation. The skin can be cleaned, numbed and a scalpel can be used to remove a sample. Pathologists can then look at the tissue and tell me what it is. Genital warts are usually pretty easy to treat with medication or surgical removal. The pathologists also help to make sure that no advanced pre-cancer or cancer is present in the lesion. #ilovepathologists

Molluscum Contagiosum

This is caused by another virus that is transmitted by skin contact and can lead to painless fleshy growths. Biopsies are often necessary to confirm this diagnosis, and these can also be removed in the office by a gynecologist or a dermatologist. In the genital region, these often are sexually transmitted, but they can be present on any part of the body and passed from any skin-to-skin contact. Hand washing is extremely important when touching the genital region. SIDEBAR: LADIES, PLEASE stop showing me your new lumps or bumps by touching your genital region, then without any involvement of soap and water, touching your head, your phone, the doorknobs in my office, etc. Just because you are comfortable with your body, doesn't mean you need to spread that love all around the office. Wash your hands or just tell me where your area of concern is, and let me find it without you bare-finger touching the area and carrying on like it's a regular day. I wash my hands like I have OCD and wear gloves for a reason. I don't want my pen that you want to borrow to be an unsuspecting vessel for your personal places.

Moles

A pigmented mole that has any irregularity or is changing in any way should be evaluated for possible melanoma or any other abnormality. If you have had that same pigmented or non-pigmented mole forever and it never has changed, leave that bad boy alone. It isn't bothering anybody. If it really bothers you, it can be removed, but the likelihood of danger in a painless stable lesion is slim to none.

Genital Herpes

An initial herpes outbreak is usually the cause of significant localized pain as well as swollen, tender inguinal lymph nodes for days to weeks. Recurrences are usually not as bad. They can cause more mild tenderness, small lesions, itching or tingling. This is where that mirror can come into play. When I diagnose a person with herpes who is having an outbreak but didn't know she even had the disease, it is usually someone who thinks she just has a yeast infection or "scratched" herself, but never looked down there to see if there was any localized skin break. If you see a small cluster of clear vesicles, or even a single tender pimple like structure or open sore, it is probably worth seeing your gynecologist right away to check it out and run some tests.

Candidiasis

If you are itching and nothing seems to help, the cause may be yeast. Itching is the hallmark. Abnormal smell is an uncommon symptom. Some can develop small bumps from yeast. I don't fault a woman for trying an over the counter yeast medication prior to coming in to see her gynecologist. I am not a huge fan of the 1-day over the counter meds. I like a 3-day or longer treatment for the best possible chance of complete treatment.

Syphilis

Though it sounds like a diagnosis of yesteryear, it is not. Syphilis is still an STD that is alive and well. If you have a painless ulcerated lesion that is not easily explained (how does one easily explain that?) or swollen lymph nodes without a good cause (what is a good cause for swollen lymph nodes?), call your Gyne and come in for testing. This lesion could last for 3-6 weeks without treatment but then resolve. That, unfortunately, is the first of the 3 stages of syphilis. The good news is that this disease is curable with antibiotics, but the diagnosis needs to be made first.

Tick Bite

You would be surprised how easy it is to not realize that you have a tick that has bitten and burrowed into your skin. This can cause a sore lesion with a black scab-like thing in the middle. That "thing" will have legs at first, but then the legs will burrow under the skin along with the head. The problem with pulling ticks out on your own is that the head can break off and stay in your skin. The head needs to be removed to avoid infection and any other tick-bite repercussions need to be monitored. You won't find me camping again after it happened to me in elementary school that ONE GOOD TIME. One got me on my torso by my bottom rib. Talk about wanting to jump up out of your OWN SKIN. Ughhhh (as I shake in my own seat almost three decades later).

Bartholin Gland cyst or abscess

This is a painful enlargement of the labia on one side or the other caused by either a blocked, or blocked and infected Bartholin gland. With a mirror, the one side of the labia will appear significantly swollen and asymmetric. These can sometimes resolve on their own with warm compresses and warm baths. Sometimes, they need to be drained by a doctor and antibiotics may be necessary. Again, PUT THE NEEDLE DOWN. In extreme and recurrent cases, a small catheter needs to be placed inside of the cyst/abscess to allow for complete drainage. Sometimes the entire gland needs to be removed. These extremes are infrequent so starting with tolerable heat twice daily down below is a great first step to try to stop these in their tracks.

If you are looking for more details, feel free to take your curiosity back to Google. Enter the "Images" tab at your own risk. Better for you to stick with this general guideline and call your doctor for an ASAP appointment if you need further evaluation of your specific issue. Don't worry, you can't gross me out. I'm a GYNECOLOGIST.

Tampon

Does toxic shock syndrome (TSS) still exist? I've never seen it. Now don't go leaving your tampons in the vagina indefinitely. Don't test those waters. Just because we don't often see toxic shock syndrome doesn't mean it can't happen. TSS is still a "thing."

On the subject of tampons staying in the vagina, I can't get through a book, authored by a gynecologist, without discussing retained tampons. Almost always the lady who thinks she left a tampon in her vagina has not. The lady who says, "I thought I inserted a tampon this morning, but I can't find it, and I think it is still there," almost never has one there. I don't know what happened to it. Maybe you never inserted it. Maybe it fell out. Maybe you pushed it out with a big bowel movement. Maybe you removed it and don't remember. I do a lot of things that I don't remember. Hell,

I have written entire sections of this book and don't remember when it happened. What I can do is tell you that it isn't there anymore. I know this because your vagina is not a never-ending abyss.

As I hope you learned in the anatomy section, the vagina has a beginning and an end. At the top of the vagina is the cervix or the vaginal cuff if you've had a hysterectomy. (Why you would need a tampon without a uterus or cervix? I will never understand—go see your doctor, please.) If you can touch your cervix, which has the texture of the end of your nose, you have felt the whole thing. If you don't feel a tampon in there, there isn't one in the vagina. A tampon cannot fit in your urethra, the place where urine comes out, and a tampon in the anus warrants some serious explanation.

The women who DO have retained tampons are the ones who come in saying that they have noticed a pungent vaginal odor and/or irritation that they can't get rid of. This odor triumphs over the most extensive bath or shower and sometimes is worse with sex. (Gag! There is an old tampon in your vagina, and you are doing "it" like it's just a regular day.) Few things in this world make me cringe or nauseous. If you read Chapter 4, that contains all of the things that make my gynecologist skin feel creepy crawly; item #10 is a retained tampon. A woman with an extremely foul discharge whose last period was 1-3 weeks ago gets my heart racing. I suck it up, put on my big girl panties and retrieve that cotton bomb like a boss. I also double bag it and ask my ladies to take it out to the street trash because it will stink up the exam room worse than a dirty diaper. Once removed, whatever vaginal discharge that was present will either resolve spontaneously, or a bacterial vaginosis may be present and require treatment.

The take-home message here is that if you smell something foul, and a retained tampon is even the slightest of possibilities, a single finger to the cervix can confirm or deny the presence of this slimy stowaway before it leads to that TSS that none of us have ever seen but don't want to tempt. When in doubt, I'm happy to check it out.

Thyroid

Ahh, my arch endocrine nemesis. The thyroid is an organ that causes so much trouble in the gynecologic world, but is so, so far away. It is in your NECK, but it CONTROLS YOUR PERIOD? What?

Okay, that's not the only thing that your thyroid is responsible for, and to be fair, your brain controls your period too. If the thyroid is overactive or underactive, the first thing that you will likely notice is a change in your menstrual cycle. Other symptoms of thyroid disease are weight changes, skin changes, hair changes, intolerance to heat or cold and neck swelling. Thyroid enlargement, known as a goiter, is not always present with thyroid abnormalities, and conversely, a woman can have a goiter without having any abnormality in thyroid function. Nonetheless, neck enlargement, asymmetry or a mass should be evaluated by a doctor.

Thyroid cancer is rare, but it does affect women more often than men and women in their mid-40s to 50s. I have diagnosed a number of goiters and nodules in my career. I usually send women for imaging if I see an enlargement or asymmetry in their neck. If you suspect an issue, see your doctor right away or ask your internal medicine doctor to examine you every year.

This feels like a good time for a sidebar. Actually, with me, it is always a good time for a sidebar. I am a Gynecologist, right? Right. I am considered a primary care physician. However, in a major metropolitan city like Chicago, a person doesn't need to wear every hat. Hell, every hat doesn't fit on every head. I know everything that I need to know about your and my vaginas. I can't say the same for your earache, your sinus infection or your plantar fasciitis. What am I saying? I am saying that you can put me or your gynecologist down as your PCP, but if you walk through my door complaining about your pinky toe, I'll send you to see a "generalist," aka "general practitioner," aka "internist," aka "internal medicine doctor," who was trained to evaluate and treat your whole body from head to pinky-toe. More on doctor roles in the Obstetrician section.

Thongs

I hate thongs. Some may think that they are sexy. Some think they are comfortable. As a matter of opinion, comfortable, they are not. Sexy? All I have to say about that is that I know one piece of clothing that only one person is going to catch me in, and I bear his name and his ring, and I will only be wearing said item for a brief pre-game show before the "kick-off." Too much? Really? We've been talking about YOUR vaginas all book. Lighten up.

I grew up thinking that you wear thongs to avoid panty lines in tight pants or skirts. I have a way better vag-happy solution for that issue: boxers or boxer briefs. I don't have an underwear line issue unless I wear pants that are too tight with boxers that are too loose. As long as I have the proper boxer to pant tightness ratio, I'll be fine and line-free.

Grandma Goodall taught me that my lady parts need to breathe. On one visit during adolescence to her house in West Virginia, I forgot to pack underwear. Our trip to the local department store to pick up a pack sparked a conversation that ultimately ended up with me disclosing the fact that I sleep in my panties. Granny said I shouldn't. Whaaaa? The concept was as foreign as a baby going without a diaper. Short of bath time, underwear was an all-of-the-time type of thing. This revelation didn't come full circle until my college years when I realized that I could simulate the freedom, the breathability, and lack of wedgie with boxers. AND boxers do not leave a panty line either! A good boxer brief's line is right sub-cheek and barely noticeable. If you see that, you are looking way too hard.

Boxers and boxer briefs are everything to me. I just don't find a perpetual thong wedgie fun at all. Not at all. I wear boxers under dresses, skirts, pants, capris and shorts. My swimsuits even have boyshorts. It could have to do with my hip/butt complex, but even regular panties have a tendency to ride their way up into my shadies (where the sun don't shine, get it?) I only wear panties if I need a liner for the occasional spotting, and I am not a period lover so that need arises very infrequently.

Ohh, maybe I should make a brand of ladies boxers and boxer briefs, since all of mine are men's, and when my momma takes pity on me and puts away our laundry, she puts my undies with my husband's boxers, leaving him with crushed jewels because my underwear are significantly smaller than his. If mine were cute enough to easily differentiate, I would be able to get dressed more easily in the morning, and his "riders" would always have more freedom. #freedomriders

Let's start a revolution. Free your bottom. Burn your thong. Don't start any domestic fires though. The bathtub is not a safe place for burning anything (R.I.P. Left Eye). On second thought, just throw them away if you share my feelings. If you love your thong, more power to you. Like ladies who deliver babies without pain meds, you are stronger than I am.

Tubes

Ear tubes… no, not really. I cannot write about ear tubes in a book about vaginas. Well, I could, but I don't want to. Ear tubes are not sexy. Fallopian tubes, now those are SEXY. I am such a gynecologist. There is so much to cover.

Tubes when you don't want to get pregnant:
A permanent, yes PERMANENT, form of birth control is a tubal ligation/occlusion. This is a method of birth control that should only be tackled if you know that you know that you KNOW that you don't want any children, or any more children. Anyone who tells you that they can reverse a tubal ligation if you change your mind is likely just out to collect your money. Can a tubal reversal work? Sometimes, but your chances of it not working or increasing your chances of having an ectopic pregnancy are substantially higher. Don't have your tubes tied unless you are MORE THAN SURE. You will know that feeling when you feel it. I feel it every day.

There are a few ways to perform a tubal ligation. The most effective, least chance of failure one is the kind done during a C-section. Traditionally the tubes are isolated, tied off and a 1-2 centimeter section is removed. Now, instead of just cutting the tube, the science is moving more toward removing the entire fallopian tube because this lowers your risk of ovarian cancer. We've learned that ovarian cancer can come from the tube, not just the ovary. The idea is that if the tubes are not needed but could possibly cause trouble later in life, get rid of them. In 2017, this is just starting to become a more popular practice. Medicine evolves so quickly that in the not-too-distant future, this will either be an automatic procedure in surgery, or it will have fallen out of favor. Time will tell.

Other methods of tubal occlusion include laparoscopic burning of the tubes, clipping of the tubes, or sliding a ring over the tube. Another way to do the procedure is to hysteroscopically insert metal coils through the inside of the tubes. After this procedure, the tubes scar around the coils and occlude themselves. They close from the inside out. What is nice about the hysteroscopic procedure is that it doesn't involve major anesthesia or cutting of any kind. Laparoscopy, if you recall, involves cutting the skin. Hysteroscopy can be done in my office, with the aid of some local and oral pain medications. The downside to this form of birth control is that it is not immediately effective. Much like a vasectomy, you have to wait

175

to ensure that the procedure works. Three months of alternative birth control needs to be consistently used. Then a confirmatory test is performed to make sure that either the tubes are totally occluded or that the coils are in the right location to presume complete occlusion.

Tubes when you DO want to get pregnant:
As discussed in the Infertility section, tubes need to be open in order to get pregnant naturally. If a reasonable amount of time has elapsed with no pregnancy, I can check to see if the tubes are open. If they are not, I cannot open them, but I can know what tactics to use to help get you pregnant. Are your tubes on your team?

Let's say that open tubes are on your team working for you. Blocked/occluded tubes are neutral. You can work around them with IVF. If the tubes are full of fluid, which is called hydrosalpinx, then that is when the tubes are working against you. This often occurs as a result of a past or present STD. It becomes relevant after treatment of the infection because that fluid can sometimes prohibit normal pregnancy implantation. That fluid leaks into the uterine cavity and can basically poison any attempt at conception. When discovered, the tubes often have to be interrupted laparoscopically, much like the procedure for a tubal ligation. This leaves pregnancies only achievable by IVF.
Take-home message: Fallopian tubes are the conduits for pregnancy, but they are a one-way street. Once they are blocked, you should consider them blocked forever and not try to reopen them. #done

U.

UTI

Back in the Anatomy section, you hopefully learned that where you urinate is not the same place that your vagina is or the same place where you have bowel movements. A man urinates through the same hole that he ejaculates out of. For the purposes of understanding in this female book, men pee out of their vaginas. We, however, do not. Our place of urination is different from the vaginal entrance, though they are only a few millimeters apart.

"Doc, I think I have a urinary tract infection."

"Why do you say that, Avey?"

"Because (choose the best option)

1. my vagina itches."

2. I have more discharge."

3. it burns when I urinate; and/or I am urinating way more frequently than normal, and the amounts are small; and/or I am having pain in my back and have a fever; and/or I have seen blood in my urine and I am not on my period; and/or my urine smells foul and pungent."

The answer is 3, Jim. No, you don't need to have all of those to possibly have a UTI, but at least one or two symptoms make the diagnosis more likely. If you have worsening back pain and what feels like a fever, you may need IV antibiotics.

It is important for a woman to get her urine tested if she thinks she has a urinary tract infection, especially if symptoms seem frequent or recurrent. The reason is that, for one, symptoms of a UTI aren't always a UTI. The second reason is that antibiotic resistance is a "thing." Antibiotic resistance is where a bacteria learns how to not die when exposed to an antibiotic. Say that you are used to using a certain antibiotic to kill a certain bacteria. If that bacteria outsmarts you, you will need a different antibiotic to kill it. The only way to know if the bacteria is smarter than your antibiotic is to check exactly which bacteria is causing the infection with a culture and check its susceptibility to various antibiotics. Otherwise, you could be treating and killing some bacteria but not all, and those that remain can have more bacteria babies, and then here you are infected again.

If possible, give a urine sample to be sent for urinalysis (checking for signs of a stone, bacterial by-products or blood) and culture. If there are enough signs of an infection, I usually start antibiotics right away. Then in the days that it takes to get the culture results back, hopefully, the infection is being treated. The results can then be used to guide further treatment of the present infection or validate and guide the treatment of future UTI symptoms.

Cranberry juice? I wouldn't overdo it. There are so much sugar and bladder irritants in cranberry juice, I don't consider this a natural treatment for urinary tract infections. If you want to go cranberry, go cranberry pills, or D-mannose. I don't mind those if they work for you. D-Mannose is a supplement used to prevent and treat urinary tract infections. I don't recommend this as a treatment, primarily because if it doesn't work, a kidney infection could develop, and kidney infections are real. By real, I mean REAL DANGEROUS. Anyway, D-mannose was brought to my attention by one of my patients because she suffered from recurrent UTIs. She wiped from front to back, urinated after sex, drank a lot of water, and still had to deal with UTIs every 1-2 months. Since trying D-mannose, she said the frequency dropped substantially.

D-mannose is a natural molecule that is found in cranberries, apples and some other fruits. It is the active ingredient in cranberries, minus the sugar that usually accompanies cranberry products like juice. Sugar is not an infection's best friend so being able to consume the active ingredient without the sugar is best. The molecule has been found to reduce the ability of bacteria to adhere to the urinary tract, which is why I think that it is most useful for prevention. The bacteria don't even make it in the door, let alone have an opportunity to trash the place. Risks are relatively low with this product, especially if used as directed.

So, what of the recommendations to urinate after intercourse and wipe from front to back. Those hold true, but ultimately some women are just more susceptible than others. Being well hydrated with water, decreasing physical and emotional stress, getting sleep at night, and regular exercise can decrease a person's risk for any infection, including those of the urinary tract.

Underwear

I already gave you my full underwear rant in the Thong section. I will only add that I had a patient who once told me that it was okay if she spotted after her Pap because she wore her spotting underwear to the appointment. Her what? That moment made me so happy. Do you have spotting underwear? It made me question what other types of underwear that we as women have?

- Spotting underwear
- Period underwear
- Workout underwear
- Date night underwear
- Sleep underwear
- Mom underwear—which is probably the same as Granny

Panties
- Stretched out underwear
- My boxers
- Commando

This is so fun!

9
DR. EVERY WOMAN IS NOT PERFECT

I am so flawed, y'all, you don't even know, but you are about to. If TMI makes you nervous, first don't try to read a book written by a gynecologist about all things female. If you have made such a decision to tackle this work of literary art, you may want to skip this chapter. There's nothing hardcore here, but there really is no such thing as TMI with me.

Did I really think that I could get through my first grown-folks book (Yay!) without sharing something personal about myself? It's only fair to dish about myself since I get up close and personal with women's most personal spaces multiple times every day. I am very nosey and like to ask the tough questions too: "Why did you get divorced? How did you meet him? What is your boss talking about? Your momma told you what?" I'm like a Gyne Barbara Walters or, better yet, a Gyne Oprah Winfrey. I tell ladies at our first meeting that I like to be nosey, and they don't have to answer all of my questions. They usually respond by saying something to the effect of, "There is no need to hold back. It doesn't get much more personal than a Gyne exam." True.

Anyway, back to my deepest darkest secrets. In undergrad, I was debt-free but too broke to appreciate it. Now after practicing medicine for over a decade, I am so broke that I can't see straight sometimes (through my tears that is). HOW SWAY? #KanyeWest. I'll tell you. I was fortunate to not have student loans in college. I only had to take them out for medical school. To the tune of $250,000.00. When you spend four years in medical school and have to borrow that kind of money, you don't think much of it because you are about to be a doctor, right?

Then I spent four years in residency, making about $30,000 per year, which paid for my husband and me to live. We were pleasantly surprised with my oldest son at the conclusion of my first year in residency. I love my son, but kids cost money. Between living and childcare, we had to defer making payments to our student loans. Now, nine years later, we have grown our family with two more children. What sometimes happens when you wait to have kids is that you limit your possibilities of being able to have them based on age and biology. You may have to pay more for them with assisted reproductive technologies or adoption. What we did was have them before we could really afford them and before we paid down some of our big student loan debt. I don't know which is better or worst.

Oh, did I mention that I met my husband in medical school? So, turn that $250,000.00 in debt to $500,000.00 in debt. But don't cry for me, we are both doctors, except that he and I spent four and seven years, respectively, in training after medical school before making any real money to pay down those loans. That allowed something called compound interest to happen. Compound interest is when the interest that is accruing on a loan is able to capitalize and shift to the principal of the loan, making it able to accrue interest. Now, my interest is collecting interest, and our payments in 2017 total almost $5000 per month and barely make a dent in the amount owed. My student loans are not tax deductible, and after you lump in private school (sorry Chicago Public Schools), a decent home, and the highest tax bracket known to man, here I stand, broke, but not broken. Oh, you think "broke" is too dramatic of a classification for a doctor? Try being over $1,000,000.00 in debt. I think that qualifies me.

Whew, I'm glad you bought this book. If this little movement goes far, I hope to not only dig myself out of a never-ending hole but set up a future for my children. I want to help others pay down student loan debt and learn how to not get into it. If I had known that $10K today is going to be $20K by the time I could pay it, I may have made different decisions about my school choice. I would love to create a foundation that gives and also lends money to students where the interest is next to nothing. That way, paying the money back is actually possible without paying double. (Like I am doing.)

If Shanice and Toni Braxton and all of these other people with big bills can live to sing another day, I want to believe that there is hope for little old me. God is my strength. Without Him, I would faint for sure.

Oh, you wanted more dirt than just my financial woes? Okay, here you go.

I did not love my pregnancies. As I desire to practice what I preach, I will spare you the detailed account of my pregnancy complications that included but were not limited to preeclampsia, cholestasis of pregnancy, a combination vacuum-forceps delivery and nausea that never seemed to relent... Oh wait, I was supposed to keep that all to myself. The good news for you is that the stuff that happened to me may have happened because of the fact that those blessed with the ability to be healthcare providers can count on having the rarest pregnancy sh%$ happen to them. It's inevitable. Be a doctor, a nurse, even a medical assistant, and you can count on something crazy during pregnancy and delivery. This paroxysmal truth also holds for the following scenarios:

The most elaborate of birth plans more often seem to result in a C-section.

The desire to have "one more baby" so that it can be a boy or girl, almost always means that you will have the opposite sex than the one that you wanted, no matter what day in what position or in what east-west-north-south direction you got down on.

What also holds true is that those with the most laid back, least controlling, not-Type A personalities often do best in pregnancy and delivery. No shade to the Type A's out there, but sometimes letting go of control works best. Pregnancy and baby delivery are unpredictable times.

If there is one thing that pregnancy and parenthood teach well, it is that you can't control everything. That doesn't mean that I think my kids should make their own way and run rampant as their freedom allows. I am not talking about parenting from an obedience perspective. I am saying that we don't know if we are having a boy or a girl. We don't know when the baby is coming (I often joke that if I could predict that, I would be a rich woman). We don't know how they will be delivered. We don't know what their personality is going to be like. We don't know what their intellect will be. We don't know what, if any, college they will go to.

These lessons of serenity begin with not knowing how long you will be nauseous, how many aches and pains along the way you will get, whether or not you will develop gestational hypertension or diabetes, how many hours of sleep you will get on a regular basis, etc.

Okay, okay, I'll share a few more deep, dark secrets.

Fun facts:

I did not learn how to properly apply lipstick until I was 35 years old. My social media lip envy made me ask my friends and colleagues what their respective secrets and tricks were to achieve the perfect lip. Sure, I could Google and YouTube the answer, but DIY has its limitations. Getting direct recommendations from friends I knew and trusted was worth more than any search engine result. Thanks to my peeps! You know who you are.

I once rode my son's scooter over a mile to my office during a Grant Park festival in Chicago. Chicago is known for its Grant Park Festivals. From the Taste of Chicago to Jazz Fest to the momentous Lallapalooza. Call me the Grinch of Grant Park because my office is in the heart of the hubbub when these various circuses come to town. I know that people like to gather and drink and wear as little clothing as possible for fun #nooffense, but I have to go to WORK.

One morning after arriving late to drop off my kids because of the growing traffic at 8 am, I was so frustrated at the thought of battling ten more blocks of traffic to get to my office that I busted out my kids' two-wheel scooter from my trunk and rode in the most awkward way possible to work with a heavy shoulder bag and my pride on display for the world. The worst part was that the city bus that I saw when I started my ridiculous journey was the same bus that glided past me two blocks before I reached my destination.

For my entire childhood, until I was practically leaving for college, that Easter candy Cadbury bunny had me thinking that rabbits make chicken noises. I really thought that it was a coincidence or poor luck that I had never heard an actual bunny go "buck buck buck buck buck..."

I had blonde hair for years. At one point I even had the look of Kelis, a popular singer in the late '90s/early 2000s who rocked a voluminous coif that had a dark base, blonde middle, and pink ends.

My awesomely independent college roommate was dying her hair red in the dorm bathroom one day (which was against the rules #sorry), and I used her leftover dye on my own blonde edges.

My third child is a baby girl with Angela Davis hair. It is big, curly and cute until it gets tangled and crazy. I need to interject a Dear White People moment. Black hair is awesome; there is no denying that fact. It could be easily inferred by our millions of styles, products and occasional challenges that we don't like it. Shea Moisture made the mistake early in 2017 of suggesting manageability challenges for black hair mean some sort of dislike or negative feelings. The opposite is true. Our hair, with various textures and lengths, can make creating different styles and looks very fun. Though I love our hair, baby girl's hair gives me a headache some days. Don't judge me if she sometimes looks crazy. I'm trying.

My last secret is that I have a last-day-of-college tattoo. I went with a friend who was getting one for a far more emotionally sentimental reason. Here I am, the supportive friend, and in the moment, I decide to commemorate my last day in undergrad with a tattoo. My intellectual mind realized that this was probably not a good long-term decision for me. After all, I didn't have a lasting cause that I wanted to immortalize. My naivety led me to ask the tattoo artist if there was such a thing as a temporary tattoo. I now know that the real answer to that question is yes. They come with a paper back and are applied using a warm damp washcloth and about 30 seconds. The answer that I received at the time was, "Yes. If you get a brown ink, it will fade away after about five years." Perfect, I thought. Then I could live in the moment, but not commit myself to a lifelong piece of art. I should have called "Bull$%#" because that dove that represented my favorite Floetry song at the time, If I Was A Bird, will be with me until I'm finally laid to rest. At least it's cute.

V.

Vaccinations

We all get our flu shots every year in my household. I was infected by the actual influenza virus once in college, and I truly thought I was dying. I literally thought it was the end. I was in the ER in New Orleans asking for my life to be saved. More than my

184

own experience with the flu, I have taken care of three women in my career who made it to the Intensive Care Unit, requiring breathing tubes to stay alive because of influenza. All three were pregnant and one of them died. None of these ladies had any prior medical conditions, and none of them were vaccinated.

Vaccines have garnered a bad reputation in the last few decades. The unsubstantiated autism argument is all too familiar. The "flu vaccines give people the flu" argument is also common. I seek to bring new light and clarity to the subject.

Vaccines are playbooks for your body. When your body encounters a new virus, it is in the form of a protein, or antigen. If that protein makes it past your mucous membranes into your body, the body has to create antibodies to attack and remove it. Imagine that you recognize a hostile intruder at your workplace. You have to tell the security office what they look like in order for the officers to find and remove them. Meanwhile, the intruder is multiplying Matrix style, but the security office is still faxing pictures and descriptions of the intruder. What if the security office knew what that Matrix agent looked like before he walked in the door? He would be arrested in the lobby and not given time to multiply and overwhelm the staff. That is what a vaccine does. It circulates posters and memos all over your body so that when Agent Smith shows up, Neo is waiting in the lobby. It's like having the other team's playbook before the big game.

Live attenuated vaccines behave differently from inactivated ones. A live attenuated vaccine is weakened so as to not cause disease and to be killed easily, but it is active enough to develop a full immune response that will teach all of your body's "troops" to fight well. It's like full pre-season training or a whole self-defense course rather than a single class or YouTube video. On the flip-side, live attenuated vaccines can cause mild viral symptoms like body aches and low-grade fevers. Inactivated, or killed viruses, are less likely to cause those symptoms, but also don't give the best-of-the-best immunity. Your body has to spar with a live vaccine.

Morbidity/mortality stats: Less than 30 years ago (1988), there were 350,000 new cases of Polio, causing crippling paralysis that occurred within hours. In 2004, there were less than 1300 cases worldwide. Influenza still kills within the United States and leads to large numbers of hospitalizations every year. A CDC article reported five million infections and three thousand deaths avoided by the flu vaccine during the 2015-2016 season.

Influenza vaccines can be given to pretty much any population. Those most at risk are the elderly, people in a household with a child under the age of two, those with compromised immune systems from HIV, diabetes, transplants, etc., and pregnant women. Adults can easily not realize that they need boosters for Tetanus (Tdap), HPV (no booster but still sometimes missed), and Measles (MMR), among others. As adults, we all make our own choices. My hope is that those choices are based on facts. Get Your Shot.

Vagina

If you are wondering what it is, back to the Anatomy section with you. If you are wondering why it itches or has an odor, check out Smell and Vaginitis. In this section, I just want to provide you with a list of things that do not belong in your vagina, as in between the labia. Why? Because someone needs this list. Here it is:

- Astringents of any kind, like alcohol or witch hazel
- Peroxide (No, really. It has been done, and I do not approve.)
- Tea Tree Oil (though containing antifungal properties) is aggressive and can easily cause irritation.
- Any commercial "pearls"
- Webs or nests of any kind.
- Anything porous. Porous stones can hold bacteria and can theoretically put you at risk for Toxic Shock Syndrome. I advise against these.

Call me old school, but let that vagina-oven clean itself and avoid any miracle tightening agents. I believe in miracles, but I pray for my vagina, I don't put prayers in it.

Vaginitis

Vaginitis means vaginal/vulvar itch and inflammation. Like the wooliest of wool sweaters. Vaginal itch can be distracting and very uncomfortable. Often women don't know how they got to be so itchy, nor do they know how to improve these symptoms. Here are some key facts about vaginitis or vaginal itching:

1. Everything that itches is not yeast.
You would be surprised how often yeast infections are blamed for personal itch but are not the actual culprit. If you want to try something before heading in to see your gynecologist, try a 3- or 7-day over-the-counter yeast medication. If no relief, further evaluation is warranted.

2. Sexually transmitted infections can sometimes itch as well.
Don't overlook that possibility if you could be at risk (by "at risk" I mean if you are having sex at all).

3. Contact with skin products and detergents can be the cause.
Avoid "fancy" things. If you are being exposed to fragrance in soaps, detergents, perfumes or even fabric softener down there, you are at risk for skin irritation. The thinner skin of the vulva is often much more susceptible to inflammation. Wash your undergarments and your other delicates (your vagina) with hypoallergenic and fragrance-free products. Stick with cotton underwear and watch those dryer sheets too.

4. Pregnancy often leads to more discharge, which can increase moisture and lead to more itching or irritation.
It's best to check with your doctor if you think you may have an infection. I personally try to be more conservative with medication during pregnancy if I don't have a definite diagnosis.

5. Itching is not always caused by infection or exposure.
Skin syndromes, some of which include precancerous changes on the skin of the vulva, can manifest as itching. This is yet another reason why paying your gynecologist a visit is important if this nagging irritation won't go away.

So how did ancient women cure yeast and similar infections without pharmacies? I imagine cavewomen in cute leaf skirts doing the itch dance as they gathered dinner. My favorite non-antibiotic remedies and symptom managers are:
• Barrier skin healing ointment: Petroleum-based ones like Aquaphor or A&D ointments work well. A&D has a very characteristic smell, FYI.
• Probiotics: Check out the Smell section which includes the

types of probiotics that have evidence supporting their effectiveness.

•   There are countless homeopathic remedies for vaginitis, but one of my favorites is boric acid suppositories. It sounds a little aggressive. After all, why would someone willingly put a capsule of acid in their vagina? Well, lactic acid is what is produced by Lactobacillus acidophilus, which is a normal and welcome resident of a healthy vagina, so there.

•   Lose a few pounds: There are multiple ways that obesity and excess weight can contribute to increased prevalence of vaginitis. Even a 5 or 10% reduction in weight can improve every aspect of health, including vaginal comfort. Decrease your sugar intake. While diabetes can be a concern if you are experiencing frequent yeast infections, many of my patients with these symptoms don't have diabetes. Even a non-diabetic woman can often find that she will have less yeast and irritation if she avoids refined sugars like white breads, pastas and, well, sugar.

There are many ways to approach discomfort in the nether regions. If you are willing to try a couple of DIYers, have at it, with caution. If you need Gyne assistance, put in that call. What I wouldn't do is just itch indefinitely. I have always said that every woman is entitled to periodic weirdness. We can't always explain why our bodies do what they do. If it doesn't go away, though, no need to suffer in silence.

Virgin

A virgin is someone who has never had penetrative intercourse. Many mothers wish virginity on their daughters. I'm sorry to tell some of you mommas, but that ship has sailed for many of your daughters. I do find it intriguing when I find someone who continues to be a virgin well into their adulthood, like into their 20s and 30s and sometimes beyond. I ask them questions. Do you want to know what women who are virgins or who have supreme sexual discretion say is their motivation? By supreme sexual discretion, I mean that they don't have sex with someone just because he is their "boyfriend." These ladies realize that boyfriends or hook-ups come and go, but the more that she shares her body, the more emotionally and physically impacted she may be in time. Shares are for social media posts, not my body.

These ladies almost never say that their reason for sparse

sexual contact is lack of information or opportunity. To the contrary, they are often very well informed about sexually transmitted diseases, and pregnancy risks. They often are very knowledgeable about their own anatomy as well. Their choices to stay virgins mostly stem from examples of healthy relationships set by family or friends, or promises made to God as their relationships with Him continue to grow. I want to emphasize that it is their relationships with God, not just their parents or siblings. They believe in their own hearts that God's Word is for a purpose and they have decided to trust him by demonstrating their obedience. It is never a completely easy and effortless decision to not have sex, but they see the benefit to their own health, both emotionally and physically, to remain abstinent.

In my limited experience, sheltering a woman completely from the world does not a virgin make. On the contrary, people with early sexual exposure that was misguided, whether by experienced yet unknowledgeable friends or inappropriate contact, isn't the recipe for healthy sexual lives either. I hope to teach my sons and daughter all about healthy choices and realistic consequences. I will let them know that I believe in God's Word, but they have to make their own choices and form their own relationship with God. Whether or not virginity is their choice, they will not be under-informed or uninformed. They won't have to "ask for a friend." They'll be the friend who the other friend asks.

W.

Warts

There is a whole section on Human Papillomavirus that tackles this subject. Warts are also discussed in the Questions section and the Things section. Pick your poison, or be fully informed and read all three sections. Or try this, READ THE WHOLE BOOK. You'll be a new woman when you are finished. I promise.

Water

Water is either a person's best friend or worst enemy. Some people love it and can't get enough. Others can't stand the taste (ironically) or can only drink it ice-cold, or with lemon, or with some other water-modifying agent. I am a consumer, but not an avid one. I have definitely had days where my kid's water bottle showed evidence of the fact that he drank more water than I did on that day.

The watery-est of water drinkers will try to get you to believe that you need to carry around a gallon pitcher with a handle and throw back two of those per day. Do that if you want to, but science speaks differently about this particular subject. From the CDC, the Institute of Medicine (IOM) set guidelines for adequate water consumption per day back in 2004. They vary slightly between men and women and by age. For women, the adequate water consumption is 2.7 liters of water per day. For men, it is 3.7 liters.

Here is the kicker, that water consumption includes food and plain water. Based on the IOM calculations, as a woman, only about 1 liter of my total water consumption usually should come from plain water. The other 66% should come from fruits and vegetables, basically water-containing foods. What that means is don't judge me for not carrying around a big Hinckley and Schmidt bottle, but do judge me if I never eat fruit, vegetables or any water containing foods.

Water intoxication is the over-hydration, or excessive water consumption, that can throw off a person's electrolytes enough to kill them. According to the American Chemistry Society, it takes about 6 liters of water consumed in a day to kill a 165-pound person. This rapid dilution of the body's sodium leads to brain swelling which can result in comas, seizures and brain herniation, causing death. It happens more than people know, sometimes in water drinking contests, sorority or fraternity hazing, or athletic training. Tell a friend.

I keep a supply of bottled water stored in my house just because of the political and spiritual times that we are in. Figuring out the food situation or long-term safety for my family could be a concern for the future. If all of the faucets turned off today and the stores closed or were abandoned, my Just-In-CASE of water will at least help us make it a few days or weeks to figure out how to survive. Or maybe it will make our demise slow and hydrated. I pray to God for the former, or that He will swing low that sweet chariot and carry us Home.

Weights

Section disclaimer: This section will contain mostly opinion and very little science, much like those who claim that vaginal weightlifting has health benefits. This section is also a little aggressive for the faint of heart. I will quote one of my favorite lines from Pitch Perfect 2, "Avert your eyes or take it all in." Here we go.

Vaginal weightlifting is the practice of putting weighted ovules in the vagina for the purpose of strengthening the pelvic floor. Getting these special muscles stronger is said to decrease prolapse and incontinence, but it's also supposed to increase the intensity of orgasms for a woman and possibly her partner. Sound great? Well, here is my problem with the whole thing.

How much weight do you use and for how long? What if you do it wrong? What if you get a Charley horse in your vag? There is no medical evidence to support this practice, and thus there is no way to standardize it. I need to know what I am recommending and what benefit I can expect from that recommendation. That information is lacking here.

If your vagina is strong enough to pull a train, what is it going to do to a penis? I imagine a good orgasm snapping that puppy or crushing it to oblivion. Would you want to get it on with Wonder Woman? Okay, bad example because she is hot. If there were a female version of The Hulk, specifically with a Hulk-ish vagina, and you had a penis, would you tap that? I'm just posing the question. No judgment out here.

I am very germaphobic when it comes to what you touch in proximity to when you last touched your vagina. I once saw a woman who put an object in her vagina that was tied to a string that was then connected to food or weights or a SURFBOARD, and all that I can think about is, when did she wash her hands after putting the object into her vagina? How much of the rope did she touch? Where did she put the thing that was in her vagina after she took it out of her vagina? WHERE DID SHE WASH HER HANDS? The vagina is not a clean place. If you think the bottom of your shoes are dirty, the vagina is just as full of bacteria. There are more bacteria there than in most places of your body. Imagine your mouth. Would you stick your finger in your mouth, then shake someone's hand? If not, why would you be all up in your vagina or vaginal area and not consider that soap and water worthy? At least use hand sanitizer!

I don't think I can support the use of vaginal weights. I am a Kegels recommender all of the way. If that isn't sufficient, pelvic floor physical therapy or surgery may be needed to control urinary incontinence or prolapse. I am not going to judge your decision, but I am also not going to put my bid in to be the judge of a vaginal bodybuilding competition, primarily because I don't want to have to touch any of the weights, scales, or ANYONE's hands.

Woke

Woke is a term used to explain gaining an understanding of what is really going on. Like if the news or media paint the world in one light, you can consider yourself Woke if you know what is happening behind the scenes. UrbanDictionary.com had a better analogy: Getting woke is like being in the Matrix and taking the red pill.

Here is the extent of my Woke-ness (#thatsnotaword): Black Lives Matter as much as your life matters. Women's rights are as important as men's rights. I miss President Barack Husain Obama and my First Lady Michelle.

Do you want more? Well, I hope that you can wake up with a warm Cup of Joe or Chai tea. This is about as deep, or Woke, as I get.

Work-Life Balance

Your guess is as good as mine on this one. You are talking to a full-time gynecologist with a husband and a bunch of kids, and here I am writing a book? And blogging? And making music videos? And with a songbook that houses some DOPE lyrics? Tag me in your posts on this subject 'cause I can use some advice.

Okay, maybe I do have a little something to say about this subject. I work a lot. I have the equivalent of a full and part-time job, with the not-so-occasional overtime. With being on call and being called in to deliver babies, I can easily put in the hours of two full-time employees. But then there is the family and the household and the kids. How do I make it work without dropping balls? I drop balls all of the time. If you are hoping to learn from a non-ball-dropper, you've come to the wrong section of this book. My take-home message to myself is that most balls bounce and can be caught for another attempt at being held. I never was good at catching, but I have the perseverance game on lock.

X.

Xavier University of Louisiana

Oh, my alma mater. An HBCU at its finest. Though I chronical some of my pivotal educational moments earlier in this book, I have to take another moment to say how amazing it is to be a product of such an esteemed institution. Xavier University, for as long as I can remember, held the record for placing the most African American students into the medical profession over any other academic institution of higher learning in this country. What a record to hold!

My friends and colleagues who are graduates of XULA will agree that it was more than a place to catapult us into medicine, dentistry, pharmacy, health sciences, hospital administration and much, much more. It was also a place to form relationships that would last a lifetime. What Norman C. Francis, the former president of Xavier did, what J.W. Carmichael, the former director of the premedical program did, what Quo Vadis Webster, the current premed program director is still doing for us as a people, warms my heart and gives me hope. Health disparities can be tackled with cultural education and sensitivity training. They can also be tackled with ethnic diversity in the medical field. I am less likely to treat that patient of color's medical problem with bias and lack of compassion if she reminds me of one of my own family members.

On that note, why is the term "person of color" better than the term "colored?" It's not that I am advocating for the resurgence of the term colored or anything. In fact, I will proverbially knock you out (proverbially because I can't fight, but will fake it; I am from Chicago) if you call me colored. It just seems like the two terms at face value seem so similar. If I tell you not to call me a bitch, could you instead call me "person of bitch-like tendencies?" If you walked up to me with a tour guide crowd and said, "Now here is a person with bitch-like tendencies," I would most certainly play Queen Latifah's U.N.I.T.Y. in my head and "punch [you] dead in [your] eye, WHO YOU CALLIN' A B..." I sound so big and bad. Meanwhile, when my kids come home reporting any semblance of a school altercation, I am the first one saying "did you alert the teacher?" I'm all talk.

Back to the subject, AS A XAVIERITE! #1925Society

X-ray

In a society where so many professionals travel regularly for work, I am often asked if it is safe to go through airport x-ray scanners. My pregnant women are especially curious about this question. Here is the data that I found about this subject. From CBSNews.com:

One scan from a typical "backscatter" security scanner might deliver 0.005 to 0.01 millirems—far, far below the 10,000 millirems that is considered the danger threshold. "There is no known risk" from being scanned, Dr. Francis Marre, former director of radiation safety at the Massachusetts Institute of Technology, tells CBS News. "It's never been demonstrated."

How do these numbers compare with an x-ray for say a suspected broken bone or dental exam? A typical chest X-ray delivers about 10 millirems. An X-ray of the hips might deliver eight times as much. That's because the bones are bigger and so require more radiation to produce good images. Conventional dental X-rays deliver considerably less—about 0.5 each; both are much more than an airport scanner.

Did you know that you are exposed to radiation from actually flying? Taking a flight from New York to Los Angeles might expose you to between 3 and 4 millirems, at least 300 to 400 times higher than the airport scanner.

Does this information make you not want to leave your house? I sure hope not. Remember, the dangerous number is 10,000. It would take a lot of flights to get to that number. You stop counting right NOW. You are fine. Stay away from nuclear bombs. That's all any of us can hope for.

Y.

Yeast

You take that curiosity back to the Candidiasis section right now. And if you are still itching after that, pick up the phone and call your doctor, or come see me. I like how I just acted like reading the section on candidiasis was somehow going to stop you from itching. How is that possible? Add this book to the list of things to NOT put in your vagina.

Z.

Zika

I dealt with this disease extensively in the Mosquito section. Not to mention the fact that you are tired of reading this book by now.

What is left? Join my following at Gyneo-bLogic.com and send me questions. These should not be super personal questions. At least act like you are asking for a friend. I will likely not respond privately to your particular question, but I will write a blog post about the topic and plan to include the new topics in the next edition of this book.

I hope that one day, this book will serve as a resource for all women from all backgrounds to understand their bodies and vaginas for miles around. I hope that this general understanding will help us to take better care of our bodies and share accurate health information with friends, family and even offspring. I do what I do because of a gynecologist of my youth, Dr. Lewanzer Lassiter, who taught me that I could spend my life helping women understand their bodies. Doing this beyond my own exam room is the dope-est thing that I can ever imagine.

I am forever grateful to each and every person who purchased this book for education and entertainment for yourself or for someone who you care about. Like with my Powerful Nia books, if one woman, at the end of this book can say that she discovered and learned more about her body, it was worth every sleepless night and every keystroke used to put this work together.

Now, this is why your vagina smells like popcorn...

ACKNOWLEDGMENTS

I give honor to God, who is the head of my life. (Gotta start there.) I love you, Ed. You keep me grounded and inspire me to keep pushing. I love you more now than ever. Thank you to my kids, Eddie, Raymond and Cadence, for surviving my crazy. Crystal, Cheryce, Rahsaah and Rae Lynne, you have turned this dream into a reality. For that, I am forever grateful. Jaiva and Amber, thank you both. Y'all don't even realize how much your belief in me has grown my belief in myself. Marcia, you have helped me believe that I can take this thing by storm. I appreciate the fact that you don't let me doubt myself. Mom and Dad, you relieve the stress that I don't even know that I have. You pick up my slack. You are my village. Paris, you polished this diamond in the rough. It sparkles brighter and gained some carats because of you. Shelly, my sister from another mister, I love you. Thank you for lifting me up when I am down.

To everyone else, thank you for taking the time to go on this journey with me. Issa Rae, I'm awkward too, and you make me proud of it. Luvvie, you are welcome to judge me and my vagina. Shonda, I like Dove. Oprah, ask me anything and I'll tell you. Ellen, I wrote a song about it. If you'd like to hear it, invite me to your show! Michelle, forever my First Lady, Chicago's Finest, can I help you take over the world? We can educate and empower the next generation together. What do you say?

Okay, I'm done. ;-)

ABOUT THE AUTHOR

Dr. Wendy Goodall McDonald, FACOG, graduated from Northwestern University Feinberg School of Medicine and is in practice at Women's Health Consulting, IL, LLC and Prentice Women's Hospital in Chicago, Illinois.

Also known as Dr. Every Woman, Dr. Wendy is the founder and Editor-in-chief of The Gyneco-blogic, a health blog that combines education and fun. She also doubles as an author, singer, and rapper, rising as the Weird Al of women's health.

Dr. Wendy has graced the pages of Essence, PopSugar, Tonic Vice, Parents, Romper, Healthline and Self to name a few. She has made regular appearances on The Jam TV Show on WCIU and has been seen Chicago Tonight on WTTW. From Refinery29 to BlackDoctor.org, she is a rising medical influencer across all social media platforms including Instagram, Twitter, Facebook and YouTube under the keyword, @dreverywoman.

INDEX

Made in the USA
Columbia, SC
02 March 2020

88610058R00126